ACTIVATE YOUR IMMUNE SYSTEM

NATURAL SUBSTANCE
PROVIDES ULTIMATE SUPPORT

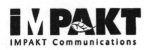

IMPAKT Communications

ACTIVATE YOUR IMMUNE SYSTEM

NATURAL SUBSTANCE PROVIDES ULTIMATE SUPPORT

by

Leonid Ber, M.D.

&

Karolyn A. Gazella

Foreword by Ray Sahelian, M.D.

Published by:
IMPAKT Communications, Inc.
P.O. Box 12496
Green Bay, WI 54307-2496
E-mail: impakt@dct.com
Fax: (920) 434-8884
www.impakt.com

Dedication

This book is dedicated to those who suffer and struggle with illness. May you find health, happiness, and most of all, peace.

General Acknowledgements

We would like to acknowledge the hard work and determination of the many gifted scientists involved with beta-glucan research. We are also grateful to all healthcare practitioners who've had the courage to ask difficult questions. Your contribution to the health of this nation is greatly appreciated.

We would also like to thank the people of the ImmuDyne Corporation for their commitment to quality products and innovative research, as well as everyone at IMPAKT Communications for their contribution to this important project. A special thanks to this book's designer, Linda Selsmeyer, and our talented editor, Frances FitzGerald.

Most of all, we would like to thank you, the reader, for your devotion to health and your willingness to consider new ideas.

Dr. Leonid Ber's Acknowledgements

I would like to thank my parents, who inspired me to choose the medical profession. Special thanks to Dr. Ludmila Afanasyeva, who "injected" me with the bug of hematology, and also Dr. Phil Wyde, Dr. Robert Nakamura, and Dr. Peter Mansell for their wise mentorship. I am also thankful to my patients, who taught me a great deal about immunology, and all the people who knowingly and unknowingly, have been guiding me through my life. Finally, special thanks to Karolyn Gazella, whose enthusiasm, devotion, and professionalism mean a lot to me.

Karolyn Gazella's Acknowledgements

I would like to thank Dr. Ber. Your hard work, commitment, and compassion do not go unnoticed. Thank you also for your technical direction on this project. I would like to also recognize the three most influential people in my life: First and foremost, my Mom, who died of cancer on January 6, 1995. What an incredible role model you were for me! Second, my sister Kathi. Your strength and unconditional love and support is appreciated so much. Finally, Maria, who has shown me true happiness. Thanks so much for your positive influence on my life and my work.

Foreword

I went through the normal process of medical education and residency, just like all medical students. We were taught about the immune system, how T-cells worked, the role of the spleen and thymus gland, and many of the intricate details of this complicated system. But, I don't recall ever being taught how to improve the immune system. It was always implied that if you left it alone, the immune system would work as well as it potentially could. There was no reason to think that any nutritional manipulation, or other modalities, could influence it. I remember asking my professor one day if there were any dietary, lifestyle, or nutritional changes one could make to boost the fighting power of immune cells. He just gave me a blank stare as if this was the first time he had ever even entertained this thought.

As I continued my medical education, I fell into the traditional medical trap of thinking that a specific antibiotic or antiviral or antiparasitic medicine was the only option in treating infectious diseases. Although these medicines have successfully treated many of the infections that had previously incapacitated or killed countless individuals, they are not the only answer. Many individuals who are afflicted with an infectious agent, or have cancer, usually have a weak immune system. Instead of just destroying the germ or the cancer cells, why not find ways to stimulate the immune system so it can effectively destroy undesirable intruders or cancerous growths?

Traditional medicine has advanced by leaps and bounds in certain areas. However, it is still in the Middle Ages when it comes to incorporating nutritional and immune-boosting approaches to its medical armamentarium.

On the other hand, we're living in an exciting age: Consumers are demanding that their doctors keep up with natural approaches and alternatives to toxic drugs. The healthcare revolution has begun!

Reading *Activate Your Immune System* will start you on the path to exploring the fascinating field of immune improvement. Together, Leonid Ber, M.D., and Karolyn A. Gazella provide an interesting perspective on some of the different ways to enhance immune function.

—Ray Sahelian, M.D.
Director, Longevity Research Center, Marina Del Rey, CA
best-selling author of books on 5-HTP, kava, DHEA,
creatine, St. John's wort, coQ10, glucosamine,
pregnenolone, and saw palmetto

Contents

Introduction

First things first

Your immune system holds the key to optimum health. It determines if you will get the flu, how long your allergy symptoms will last, and even if you will succumb to the ravages of cancer or AIDS. In large part, your immune system will dictate how you live and how you will die.

The immune system has a lot of responsibility and it becomes even more challenging in today's society. Illnesses that result from a weakened immune system continue to increase dramatically. Cancer, which is presently the most expensive and most feared disease of our time, is expected to surpass heart disease as our number one killer disease within the next few years. And it is understood that cancer cannot thrive within the confines of a strong, healthy immune system.

An immune system functioning at peak performance is also able to protect us against viruses, bacteria, yeast, fungi, parasites, and a host of toxins. If your immune system is not up to the challenge, these toxins can make you sick. The immune system has the power, it has the system and it has the players. But the task is still daunting. Consider this:

○ The overall incidence of cancer has increased by 44 percent since 1950, with breast cancer up 60 percent and prostate cancer up an amazing 100 percent.

1

○ It is estimated that 25 percent to 50 percent of the American population suffers from allergies.

○ We live in a toxic world. At least 20,000 of the 70,000 known chemicals we are continually exposed to have been proven to cause cancer. America sprays 1.2 billion pounds of pesticides on the foods we eat, while nine million pounds of antibiotics are pumped into our meat and poultry supply. Every year, 90 billion pounds of toxic waste are dumped into 55,000 sites throughout the United States.

○ Artificial colors, flavors, and preservatives are key ingredients in the increasingly popular "convenient foods" that line the shelves in grocery stores. We are discovering the long-term damage these processed foods can have on our health. Recently, Harvard-trained researcher Kilmer S. McCully, M.D., confirmed that food processing and preservatives cause heart disease by creating vitamin deficiencies of folic acid and vitamins B_6 and B_{12} thereby raising homocysteine levels in the body. Homocysteine is a non-essential toxic amino acid that leads to heart disease. Dr. McCully says he will soon be able to prove the connection between food processing and cancer as well. This will firmly establish that consumption of these foods can lead to a weakened immune system.

○ Resistance to antibiotics is becoming a very real concern. "The age of antibiotics is fast coming to a close," writes Michael Weiner, Ph.D., in his book, *Maximum Immunity*. "Because of their great numbers, viruses and bacteria have quickly evolved resistant strains for almost every major man-made pharmaceutical."

It's easy to see why the immune system has its work cut out for it. Protecting us from illness is no easy task.

"With the increasing levels of carcinogens in our environment, our bodies' demand for effective immune elimination of newly formed cancer cells is at an all-time high, and based on the increasing incidence of cancer, more and more of us are failing to meet the challenge," explains Joseph Pizzorno, N.D., president of Bastyr University and author of *Total Wellness*. "Another 20th-century problem is the growing number of bacteria that have become resistant or immune to the available antibiotics. Establishing and maintaining an effective immune system has never been more important."

Childhood ear infections are a prime example of the importance of an immune system response and the overuse of antibiotics. While studies indicate that 90 percent of all ear infections heal entirely on their own without antibiotic treatment, prescription antibiotics continue to be some of the most popular drugs available. According to author and clinician Mary Ann Block, D.O., giving antibiotics early during an ear infection is likely to cause more recurrences and lead to more bacterial resistance.

"Even if the antibiotic does not help us get well any faster, there is a tendency to want that antibiotic prescription anyway," explains Dr. Block. "This attitude may have actually put our future health in jeopardy."

It's up to our immune systems to help protect us from the new, "super" germs being created through antibiotic resistance. Some of the simple bacteria that were easily treated with a commonly prescribed antibiotic no longer respond. Other infectious bacteria, such as tuberculosis—once thought to be under control—are recently resurfacing and are more challenging to treat than ever before. And the issue of bacterial resistance is just one of the many serious health concerns the body's immune system has to deal with.

It's clear that keeping the immune system healthy and strong should be our first priority if we are to avoid disease and achieve optimum health. How we age and the quality of our life depend largely on the health of our immune system.

Unhealthy health care

Fortunately, how we view health care has undergone a critical shift over the past several years. Consumers, as well as many medical doctors, are realizing we can no longer depend upon heroic measures after a disease has taken hold—especially diseases associated with a weakened immune system. Successful health care is based on the ability to prevent disease and stimulate the body's healing powers.

"The result of human evolution is that our bodies have become finely tuned instruments that have the capability of fighting against almost every kind of invading organism or every internal disturbance," according to Dr. Weiner. "...it is no longer valuable simply to attack the disease without building up the strength of the immune system first."

Recognizing that the power lies within us and that we can activate and enhance that power is the first step toward successful disease prevention and treatment. This does not mean we should turn our backs on conventional medicine. Conventional, often called allopathic, medicine has much to offer us. A truly successful healthcare system provides a comprehensive treatment and prevention plan. It does not have to be an either/or proposition.

Common sense suggests that you must first take the least toxic, most effective route possible. And by reading this book, you will discover a new way to activate the power of your immune system. You will discover the incredible benefits of a natural compound known as beta-1,3-D-glucan. This will help you prevent illness and may provide the perfect complement to an existing treatment plan.

But first, a word of caution: If you are experiencing symptoms of a compromised immune system, self-diagnosis is not advised. Please see a qualified physician for a professional diagnosis and treatment options. The information in this book is educational only. It is not intended to help diagnose or treat illness.

Congratulations!

By reading this book, you are taking an important step toward developing your ultimate immune system potential. You are making a commitment to your health—your most important and irreplaceable asset.

This book will explain how you can stimulate a positive immune system response. You will discover how an impressive scientific breakthrough can safely and naturally activate your immune system. You will be sure to get all of your questions answered in chapter four. Most importantly, you will be given the knowledge you need to protect against cancer, AIDS, allergies, chronic colds and flu, candidiasis, and much more.

But first, let's unlock the mystery of the human immune system. Discover your own power to be healthy. It exists within each one of us

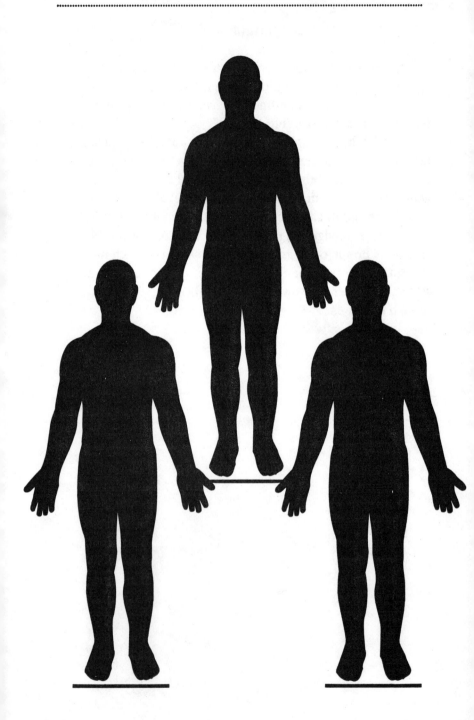

Chapter One

Recognize the power

The human immune system is an amazing internal computer, comprised of trillions of cells working together to accomplish the same goal—to keep us healthy! It has been compared to an army, fighting our battles and protecting us from the enemy.

We like to think of it as the ultimate team effort, where all the players know their exact responsibilities and carry out their tasks when called upon. Ideally, it's a smooth-running system built on timing, persistence, and strength.

Around the clock, our immune system team works to protect us against illness. The team includes a complex array of organs, tissues, fluids, and cells carrying out a sophisticated, health-promoting strategy.

"The trillions of specialized warriors in our immune system are on 24-hour duty, vigilantly destroying and mopping up virus, bacteria, yeast, tumor cells, and toxins..." explains cancer expert Patrick Quillin, Ph.D., in his best-selling book, *Beating Cancer with Nutrition.* "The crucial missing link in most cancer therapy is stimulating the patient's own healing abilities."

Dr. Quillin explains that even the best medical equipment can't detect one billion cancer cells circulating throughout your body. "Imagine leaving behind only one billion dandelion seeds on your lawn after you thought you got them all," he explains. The 20 trillion cells that make up the immune system are responsible for eliminating cancer cells or other toxins in your body.

Primarily, the body utilizes non-specific, cell-mediated immunity when it makes its first strike. The goal of cell-mediated immunity is to attack the invader immediately and not allow it to take hold, or destroy it as quickly as possible if it has taken hold. Cell-mediated immunity provides us with vital protection against cancer and allergic reactions. It also helps us resist a variety of infections.

The effectiveness of the immune system depends on several key components. Let's become familiar with some important immune system terminology.

Antigens. Antigens are foreign molecules that represent "non-self" (i.e., anything the immune system views as "not belonging"). An antigen is a portion of a cell, a molecule that is a part of something that can and does destroy healthy cells. Examples include viruses, bacteria, fungi, pollen, harmful chemicals, undigested food proteins, and cancer cells.

Antibodies. The B-cells produce antibodies to kill antigens. The antibody can disable bacteria, help scavenger cells eat antigens, and block viruses from entering healthy cells.

B-cells. These cells circulate throughout the body and originate in bone marrow, lymph nodes, and spleen. When they recognize an antigen, they grow larger and spew antibodies to help eliminate the antigen. These antibodies are particularly effective against bacteria and viruses.

Cytokines. The cells within the immune system communicate with each other by using protein messengers called cytokines.

T-cells. These cells mature in the thymus gland and then circulate throughout the immune system. T-cells serve many important functions, including informing other cells about antigens, fighting antigens directly, and regulating the immune response. T-cells also include natural killer cells that kill antigens.

Thymus. This gland is locate
behind the breast bone. This is wl
grow stronger.

Spleen. This organ is located
domen. In the spleen, many key
system collaborate and interact, i

Lymph nodes. These vital imr
located in the neck, armpits, gro
heart, and around the digestive or
from the tissues that help remove antigens from the ......

Bone marrow. This is the soft material that fills the bone
cavity in the long bones of the arms and legs. B-cells are produced in the bone marrow, as well as some T-cells and
macrophages.

Macrophages. These cells are produced in the bone marrow and circulate throughout the body. Macrophages engulf
and digest (i.e., "eat") antigens. They also help T-cells recognize antigens for future encounters.

Because the macrophage is such a critical component of the
immune system, it's important to fully understand its action.

The mighty macrophage

If you were in a pie-eating contest, you'd want the mighty
macrophage on your side. After all, macrophage literally
means "big eater." Like a hungry octopus, the macrophage
extends its "arms" to pull in infectious invaders, eating and
destroying them.

In addition to having a huge appetite for toxins,
macrophages play an essential role in the initiation and maintenance of the immune response. Once macrophages become
activated, a chain reaction occurs that mobilizes and amplifies
the entire immune system.

"...macrophages patrol, scavenge, attack, and destroy
invaders, send for help, and remove debris," according to the
editors of Time-Life Books in *The Defending Army: Journey*

and Body. "Their technique for disposing of
erial is simple but dramatic: They consume it."
ocess takes place in our bodies billions of times
! A healthy immune system has billions of macro-
s working on the job non-stop.

Let's pause for a moment to visualize this: Billions of
macrophages eating toxins billions of times each day. How
does this equate to time? Well, one million equals 12 days
worth of seconds. One billion equals 32 *years* of seconds. And
one trillion (keeping in mind that there are actually trillions
of cells in the human body) equals 32,000 years of seconds.
That's an enormous amount of activity and power!

"It seems the more the macrophage eats, the more it gets
turned on to the job," according to Ellen Michaud, Alice
Feinstein, and the editors of *Prevention* Magazine in their book
Fighting Disease: The Complete Guide to Natural Immune Power.
"Once they arrive on the scene, they liven up. They move faster,
seemingly delighted with the microbial banquet."

Eating isn't the only task at which the macrophage excels.
It also makes antigens easily recognizable to commander
T-cells. Because of this function, the immune system is ready
and waiting the next time the same antigen enters the body.

According to *Taber's* medical dictionary, macrophages "serve
as the major scavengers of the blood, clearing it of abnormal
or old cells and cellular debris..." Although mature
macrophages are found in virtually all body tissues, *Taber's*
tells us that macrophages are primarily found in large quantities in the spleen, lymph nodes, alveoli (tooth sockets and air
cells in the lungs), and tonsils, and they have a life span of
several months. From an evolutionary point of view, the
macrophage is the oldest and most consistently immunologi-
cally competent cell known. Macrophages are extensively
involved in:

O everyday detoxification
O intestinal flora maintenance
O protection against infections and tumors

○ removal of the body's aged, dead, and
  abnormal cells and tissues
○ general support of overall health

The macrophage is a veritable powerhouse. It can actually recognize and kill tumor cells, as well as remove foreign debris. In addition, the macrophage boosts bone marrow production of critical immune system team players.

Think of the immune system as an upside-down pyramid. At the bottom is a single cell that is usually the first to recognize and attack something that is foreign and harmful. The macrophage is that cell. Stimulating the macrophage helps produce a *balanced* response that enhances the performance of the entire pyramid. This is known as the immune cascade.

Scientists are aware that some substances (i.e., drugs) produce instant immune stimulation in certain parts of the cascade but actually shut down and interfere with other components of the cascade at the same time. This immune imbalance is a common complication of some pharmaceutical drugs, such as interferon. The key is to activate a balanced response that originates from the very roots of the cascade, the tip of the pyramid. This will utilize, not disrupt, the natural chain of command within the immune system. And it all starts with the macrophage.

Together with the other key components of the immune system, macrophages work diligently to gobble their way to our good health. In concert, the immune system team members methodically and meticulously protect us from foreign, disease-causing invaders.

But what happens when the immune system team falters? What happens when our immune system is not operating at peak performance?

Something's wrong

The power of our internal immune army is undeniable. And yet, the immune system, in all its majesty, can become vulnerable. Many factors can weaken immune function, including:

○ environmental toxins, specifically in the air and water
○ toxins in the food supply
○ poor diet (i.e., high-calorie/low-nutrient value)
○ unhealthy lifestyle habits (i.e., smoking, over consumption of alcohol, lack of exercise)
○ extended periods of stress
○ emotional aspects (i.e., lack of love or laughter)
○ genetic predisposition
○ dramatic lifestyle changes (i.e., death of a loved one, loss of a job, divorce)

In his book, *Maximum Immunity*, Dr. Weiner explains that the reason we get sick is that sometimes there is a time lapse between when the foreign "invader" enters the body and when the immune system actually destroys it. "In the interim, the pathogen {disease-producing organism} is doing its damage to the body—killing cells, making toxins, devouring nutrients and energy," he explained. Even after the immune system has the invader under control, it can still take a while for the body to rebound.

The duration and severity of the episode is largely determined by how strong our immune system was prior to the attack. If any one of the key components of the immune system is not performing satisfactorily, it can sabotage the success of the immune response. For example, if there aren't enough macrophage cells to devour the invader, the antigen can't be eliminated from the body. If the B-cells don't release sufficient antibodies to destroy the antigen, the invader will remain in our system. All factors of the immune system must be functioning properly to ensure optimum immune response.

Viruses, bacteria, and other antigens need the healthy cells in our body to survive. Without healthy cells, antigens can multiply and spread their toxic chemicals throughout the body. "When you have a viral infestation, the viruses actually take over the cells of your body to serve their own reproductive purposes," explains Dr. Weiner.

A weak immune system is unable to muster enough energy to protect the healthy cells and kill the virus. That's why we get sick.

Let's use the example of the common cold. If you're like most people, you can't get through the cold and flu season without experiencing a "bug" or two. While this may be common, it's completely unnecessary. As we have seen, a healthy immune system can eliminate the countless viruses we encounter, keeping us healthy all year long. But what if your immune system is weak?

It may begin with a seemingly harmless sneeze from a co-worker. "A sneeze reportedly explodes from the mouth and nostrils at 40 miles per hour, as opposed to the relatively gentle five miles per hour for normal breathing," according to Michaud and Feinstein. "And hitching a ride on every minute droplet expelled by that sneeze are countless homeless viruses, all hoping to encounter someone just like you."

Before you know it, you take an unconscious breath and the virus lodges at the back of your throat, warm and content. There, it begins to multiply. Your immune system sends the alarm about the new invader and tries to attack. You may get a fever, or your throat may become inflamed. It may take days for your weak immune system to build a big enough army to overtake the rapidly dividing virus. And then, just as you think you've managed to kick this virus out of your system, you get sick again. Sound familiar? Unfortunately, while a weak immune system may be able to eventually take care of the invader, it has a hard time handling new invaders shortly after the fight.

Allergies are another example of the impact a condition has on the immune system, and how the immune system

works with that condition. Millions of people suffer from irri-
tating, sometimes life-threatening allergy symptoms.

It is interesting to note that modern, common allergies are
really a fairly new phenomenon. The number of people with
allergies has risen dramatically. In fact, 100 years ago, the
word "allergy" did not even exist. In 1950, an estimated one
in seven Americans had allergies, while in 1970 there was one
in five, and in 1985, one in three.

People may be allergic to pollen, grass, mold, hay, per-
fumes, foods, food preservatives, and a variety of environmental agents. Typically, an allergic reaction is caused when
the immune system views the allergen as an antigen/toxin,
thus creating an immune response.

"Allergies can cause an amazing array of diseases, including
immune problems, arthritis, diabetes, heart disease, mental illness, and more," explains Dr. Patrick Quillin. "The reason allergies are so complicated to detect and treat is the limitless com-
binations of chemicals in the human body."

According to Dr. Quillin, allergies create an imbalanced
immune system. For this reason, it is important to control
allergies as much as possible.

"I consider allergic reactions to foods to be one of the
most important (and generally unrecognized) immune-sup-
pressing problems facing us today," explains Dr. Joseph
Pizzorno in his book, *Total Wellness*. "If immune-stimulating
foods are eaten frequently, the immune system's resources are
continually focused on the intestines. Viruses, bacteria, fungi,
and cancer cells elsewhere in the body have a great opportunity to invade and grow unchecked."

Freedom from allergies and a strong immune system go
hand in hand. In fact, allergy shots are a way to get the
immune system accustomed to the allergen. With allergies,
there is a two-fold reason to work on building a strong
immune system: to help ease the allergic response and to protect the immune system from damage that allergies can cause.

Countless examples illustrate the link between a weak immune system and the breakdown of health. Here are just a few:

○ **HIV/AIDS**—HIV infection and the AIDS virus are possibly the most profoundly intense examples of immunosuppression in disease.

○ **Candidiasis**—Chronic candida infection demonstrates how a weakened immune system can allow a fungus, namely candida, to overtake the system, resulting in many health problems including depression, food allergies, chronic fatigue syndrome and others.

○ **Diabetes**—A weakened immune system contributes to elevated blood glucose levels, which weakens the immune system even further.

○ **Stress-related diseases**—Physical and emotional stress can negatively affect the immune system. In stress-related illnesses, such as heart disease, the number of available macrophages is reduced. Consequently, there are not enough to participate in the immune response, causing further immune suppression. This also happens to athletes and others who work out extensively.

○ **Aging**—One of the primary byproducts of the aging process is decreased immunity. Many diseases of aging—such as arthritis; reduced wound-healing capacity; chronic viral, fungal, and bacterial infection; anemia; and cancer—can be linked to a weak immune system. This has led many anti-aging researchers to focus on immune-system stimulation in an effort to prolong quality of life.

The power of the immune system and its relation to optimum health cannot be denied. It determines the quality of our health. It is critical that we recognize the significance of this incredibly complex biological miracle.

Summary

Several key components of the immune system must remain healthy and strong if we are to be free of illness and disease. While these players work together to keep us healthy, the macrophage stands out as a leader in non-specific, cell-mediated immunity. The macrophage literally eats viruses, bacteria, fungi, parasites, and other antigens to eliminate them from the body. These "big eaters" then work with T-cells to "flag" the antigen so it is easily recognized for future battles.

When it's strong, the immune system has the power to keep us healthy. When it becomes weakened, our health suffers. A weakened immune system can result in chronic colds and flus, allergies, candida, accelerated aging, cancer, and other chronic, degenerative diseases.

The dance between the immune system and our outside world is obviously quite complex. Our goal is to help you discover the power that lies within you. Keeping your immune system operating at peak performance should be your number-one health goal. Let's find out just how you can do that.

Chapter Two

Unleash the power

Remember when you played team sports as a kid? Remember when your team was losing and you decided to bring out "the secret weapon"? Out steps the biggest kid in class who can run the fastest, hit the hardest, and throw the farthest. This changes the game, doesn't it?

Well, your immune system is that "big kid." It's the "secret weapon" within you.

Whether you are trying to prevent illness and maintain good health, or you are experiencing an illness and trying to develop a successful treatment plan, you need to unleash the power of your immune system. Without a strong immune system, you will at best go into extra innings, or at worst, lose the game. Our health and the quality of our lives depend on this inner secret weapon.

Fortunately, there are many things we can do to stimulate a consistent, positive immune response. Keep in mind, there's not just one answer—no magic bullet. The most successful immune system activation program involves many aspects. A complex concept such as enhanced immunity requires attention to detail in all aspects of living. While we cannot live completely "pure" lifestyles, the more frequently we make health-promoting choices, the better off our immune system will be.

Important aspects for optimum immune system function include:

○ proper diet
○ healthy lifestyle choices
○ exercise/physical activity
○ the mind/body connection
○ nutritional supplements as added "health insurance"

Let's take a closer look at each of these important immune-system components.

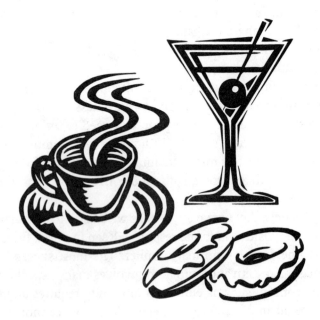

Food as the foundation

We must closely evaluate everything we put into our bodies. **Recognize that food is medicine.** The body responds to what we eat and drink, oftentimes, just as powerfully as it would if we took a drug. The dietary choices we make will either have a positive or negative impact on our health.

It is now widely accepted that the foods we eat have a direct impact on our immune system and overall health. How many times have you heard, or said, the following statements?

- "Caffeine makes me jittery."
- "Sweets give me a rush, but then I seem to crash a few hours later."
- "I get so tired after I eat a big meal."
- "I get headaches if I quit drinking coffee."
- "I just can't handle the hangovers when I drink alcohol."
- "Red wine gives me migraines."
- "I can't tolerate dairy products."
- "My child can't concentrate and gets hyper after a snack."

These are just a few of the negative "side effects" people experience with different foods or drinks. But, fortunately, there's a flip side. Let's look at some of the positive effects certain foods can have on health:

- Tomatoes have an active compound called lycopenes that have been shown in clinical studies to actually help reverse some cancers.
- Soy foods have been proven to help prevent some cancers and also ease menopausal symptoms.
- Whole grains provide sufficient amounts of fiber to help detoxify the body and help prevent some cancers.
- Vegetables are packed with vital nutrients that not only stimulate a powerful immune response, but also prevent many serious illnesses.
- Pure drinking water helps cleanse the body and is free of toxins commonly found in the public water supply.

○ Beans and legumes contain phytoestrogens, powerful compounds that can help prevent and treat many serious illnesses, including cancer.

○ Flax seeds and flaxseed oil have been shown to help prevent many cancers and other serious illnesses as well.

○ Essential fatty acids from fish and other sources have been proven to positively influence the immune system and help reduce the risk of serious illnesses such as heart disease and some cancers.

○ Herbs and herbal teas have a medicinal effect. They are used to treat many conditions such as insomnia, depression, anxiety, and compromised immune function.

Remember: Whatever we put into our bodies has an effect. The choices we make determine if the effect will be positive or negative. Fresh, unprocessed foods and pure drinking water can be our immune system's best friends.

We can also strengthen our immune systems by making healthy lifestyle choices.

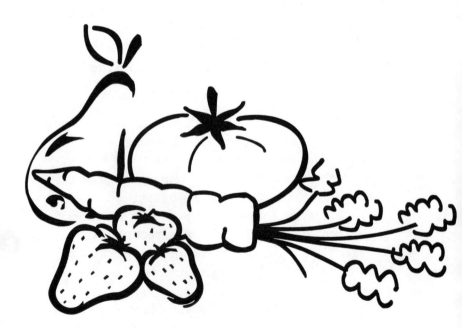

Lifestyle lessons

Each day we make choices: what to wear, where to have dinner, when to go to work, how to have fun. Just like the foods we eat, the choices we make about how we live also have a profound effect on the health of our immune system. Here are some prime examples of lifestyle choices that negatively influence the immune system:

○ **Tobacco**—Tobacco directly depletes the immune system. It saps your body of important nutrients and causes disease such as cancer and heart disease.
○ **Alcohol**—Excessive alcohol intake has been clearly linked to a variety of illnesses such as liver disease, cancer, heart disease, and others. It has also been shown to suppress immune function.
○ **Sleep deprivation**—As you rest, your immune system continues to work and regenerate itself. Insomnia can weaken the immune system and cause numerous health problems, including depression, anxiety, and other conditions.
○ **Negativity**—Some researchers have shown that a negative attitude can negatively influence immune function. Besides, it's just not fun for you *or* the people around you!
○ **Lack of love and laughter**—Not getting enough of these has a detrimental effect on immunity.

The lifestyle lessons here are clear:

○ If you smoke or chew tobacco, and want to be in good health, you need to stop!
○ Reduce or eliminate alcohol intake.
○ Listen to your body when it needs to rest and relax. If you don't, your body will get your attention with illness or disease.
○ Be positive, even when you're not feeling positive.
○ Give love and experience big "belly" laughs each day!

In addition to these, one of the most important positive lifestyle choices you can make is to exercise regularly.

Exercise is for everybody!

We often use the term "physical activity" when talking about exercise. Some people can be intimidated by the term "exercise." To exercise doesn't necessarily mean putting on spandex, buying expensive running shoes, and strapping on a Walkman every day of the week. To exercise is to increase physical activity. That can mean walking, taking the stairs instead of the elevator, parking further away from the office, or chasing your grandchildren around the back yard. The idea is to do more than you are presently doing. You will be amazed and delighted by the benefits of increased physical activity.

Many studies have confirmed that increased physical activity results in higher self-esteem, and an overall improvement in health and happiness. In addition, exercise increases strength, improves sleep quality, and helps control weight. Improving immune function is also among the long list of health benefits of regular exercise. Consistent exercise has been proven to directly benefit these conditions:

○ **Heart disease**—When combined with a healthful diet, exercise is an ideal way to unclog arteries or prevent the illnesses associated with heart disease, such as high blood pressure and elevated cholesterol levels.
○ **Menopause**—Exercise has been proven to reduce symptoms of menopause, including hot flashes.
○ **Osteoporosis**—Physical activity is the best way to keep bones healthy and strong.
○ **Depression and anxiety**—Exercise releases endorphins, important mood-enhancing chemicals that help alleviate symptoms of depression and anxiety.

○ **Cancer**—By stimulating a positive immune-system response, exercise has been shown to help prevent many cancers, including breast cancer.

○ **Diabetes**—People who exercise regularly are less likely to develop adult-onset diabetes. In addition, exercise helps diabetics control their condition better as it promotes the body's ability to lower blood glucose levels.

○ **Memory loss**—Unless there's irreversible brain damage, physical activity can invigorate and revitalize the mind. Aerobic exercise helps move blood and oxygen to all the body's organs, including the brain.

○ **Pain relief**—When you exercise, your body releases endorphins and natural cortisone, which can help relieve arthritis symptoms.

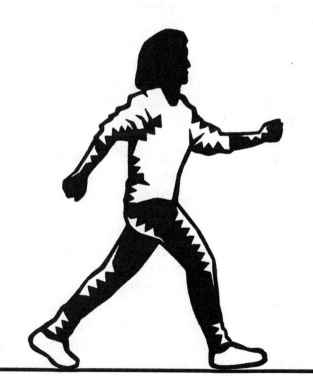

Be sure to exercise consistently. We are often asked: Which is better, to exercise once a week for an hour and a half, or exercise three times a week for 30 minutes? Hands down, the answer is to exercise three times a week for 30 minutes. Studies have even confirmed that taking two 15-minute walks during the day provides the same benefit as one 30-minute walk. The lesson here is consistency, not intensity. As you become more fit, you will, of course, want to increase your intensity to get the most out of your workout.

If you have been fairly inactive, you need to consult your physician before undertaking an exercise program.

The positive benefits of exercise are far-reaching. It's been called the most powerful medicine known. It can certainly be very economical. When you consider the return on investment, it's well worth it!

Mind/body connection

The impact the mind has on physical health is becoming better understood as researchers delve more deeply into this fascinating aspect of medicine. Unfortunately, the mind/body connection is still not getting the recognition it deserves regarding the incredible contribution it can make to our overall health.

Recently, however, some of the finest scientific institutions throughout the world are finally not only embracing mind/body medicine, they are confirming its potential through clinical studies. Candace Pert, Ph.D., with Rutgers University, is considered a premier mind/body scientist. She and many of her associates have found that the peptides and neuropeptides in the brain release endorphins. These endorphins directly affect our emotions.

"The astounding revelation is that these endorphins and other chemicals like them are found not just in the brain, but in the immune system, the endocrine system, and throughout the body," explains Dr. Pert. "When people discovered that there were endorphins in the brain that caused euphoria and pain relief, everyone could handle that. However, when they discovered they were in the immune system as well, it just didn't fit, so these findings were denied for years. The original scientists had to repeat their studies many, many times to be believed."

Now, due to the growing interest among scientists and the general public, there is even a name for the field that studies the connection between the mind and the immune system: psychoneuroimmunology. However, we'll continue to refer to it as mind/body medicine in this book.

"The immune system, like the central nervous system, has a memory and the capacity to learn," according to *Alternative Medicine: The Definitive Guide*, compiled by the Burton Goldberg Group. "Thus, it could be said that intelligence is located in literally every cell of the body, and that the traditional separation of mind and body no longer applies."

Many areas of mind/body medicine can help stimulate a positive immune response, including:

O visualization/guided imagery
O biofeedback
O spirituality/faith/prayer
O positive thinking
O self-talk and goal setting
O meditation/hypnotherapy

How many times have you gotten a bad cold or flu after a negative life event? How many times have you felt almost invincible after receiving a love letter or card? Both circumstances influence your immune system—one negatively, the other positively.

Grief, depression, fear and panic can actually suppress immune function, while laughter, love, faith, and self-acceptance will stimulate a positive immune response.

Norman Cousins, who endured serious illness, wrote about how laughter helped him regain his health. Surrounding yourself with supportive, loving people also has a powerful effect on immune function. Try to avoid "toxic" (i.e., negative or draining) relationships whenever possible.

Here are quick paraphrased reviews of two scientific studies on mind/body medicine:

1. **Love/support.** A group of men with a history of heart disease were evaluated and monitored. Detailed questionnaires revealed that the men who said they felt they had love and support from their partner, did not experience a second heart attack. In contrast, the group of men who felt they were not loved and supported by their partner, had a second and sometimes a third heart attack. The interesting aspect of this study is the connection between love and heart disease.

2. **Prayer.** A study of patients in a hospital setting demonstrated the power of prayer. Volunteers were asked to pray for a group of patients in the hospital. The volunteers were given descriptions of the people and their illnesses. There was also a "control" group of patients who were not prayed for. The patients did not know they were being prayed for. The patients' progress was monitored. Interestingly, "prayed-for" patients had significantly faster recovery times than the group who was not prayed for. While this study did not promote a particular religion, it certainly establishes an interesting perspective on a higher power and spiritual influence.

What we find most attractive about mind/body medicine is that it puts us back in control. Using mind/body medicine techniques helps us become proactive rather than reactive. This approach teaches us that true health requires emotional balance. Many psychological factors can influence our health and our healing.

Nutritional health "insurance"

Today's fast-paced society bombards us with incredible stressors, highly processed and packaged foods, environmental toxins, and enticing "convenience" foods. It can be terribly difficult to get all the essential nutrition you need from diet alone. For this reason, nutritional supplements provide important health "insurance" to help you achieve optimum health.

Keep in mind, nutritional supplements are just that—supplements to a balanced diet and lifestyle. Most of the research on nutritional supplements and the immune system have focused on the topic of free radicals and antioxidants.

Free radicals are the toxic molecules (i.e., antigens) that wage war on us. They cause damage through oxidation, similar to when a car rusts. They are in the air we breathe, the water we drink, and the foods we eat. Free radicals are also generated internally as we breathe, convert food into energy, or battle an infection. External free radicals enter the body and damage cells, potentially converting them into cancer cells or creating other debilitating diseases. When the immune system is overworked or weakened, it can't keep up with the elimination of free radicals. Fortunately, the reverse is also true. When the immune system is functioning at peak performance, free radicals don't stand a chance.

Science has discovered that certain nutrients have antioxidant activity, protecting cells from free radical damage. They can even destroy free radical cells. The *anti*-oxidation activity of these important nutrients is your immune system's "rust protectant." Researchers believe antioxidant nutrients can help prevent illness, treat degenerative diseases, and may even slow the aging process.

Antioxidants are present in many of the foods we eat. Fresh fruits and vegetables are packed with these important antioxidant nutrients. That's why it's so important to include fresh fruits and vegetables in your daily diet. Traditional, well-known antioxidants include vitamins C and E, beta-carotene, selenium, and zinc.

One of the newest, most effective antioxidants discovered is **beta-1,3-D-glucan.** This natural substance demonstrates such phenomenal potential that it is the focus of the following two chapters.

When you are looking for nutritional insurance, begin by building a strong foundation with a comprehensive multivitamin/mineral supplement. Be sure this supplement contains the traditional antioxidants, as well as other important nutrients such as B-vitamins, calcium, and magnesium. (For more information on choosing a quality multiple, refer to Karolyn Gazella's book, *Buyer Be Wise: The Consumer's Guide to Buying Quality Nutritional Supplements.*)

Countless nutritional supplements are available over-the-counter. Once you do some research and educate yourself about your options, your choices will be clearer.

An estimated one in three Americans is now using alternative health approaches. The growing interest in nutritional supplements is a direct reflection of our dissatisfaction with conventional medicine and, at times, our desperation to find optimum health. The nutritional supplement industry has escalated to more than $10 billion in sales per year, offering a variety of new and exciting options for us.

Summary

To build a strong immune system and achieve optimum health, we must utilize a comprehensive approach. The best plan includes these important components:

O healthful diet
O positive lifestyle choices
O consistent physical activity/exercise
O mind/body techniques
O nutritional supplements

With the proper support, our immune systems have the power to keep us healthy and/or alleviate disease. New substances are surfacing to assist us in this goal. One of the most promising is beta-1,3-D-glucan.

Thanks to research spanning several decades, we have access to a natural, effective substance we believe is the ultimate immune system activator—beta-1,3-D-glucan. For easier reading, we will refer to this natural compound as beta glucan; however, as you will discover, purchasing the *right* beta glucan will make all the difference in the world.

Chapter Three

The ultimate activator

Volumes have been written on the workings of the human immune system. And yet, details of how it functions on all levels remains somewhat of a mystery. At least now we have a basic understanding of how the immune system works. We know that it has the power to keep us healthy and rid the body of illness. And we know how we can best support the health of our immune system.

If only there were some simple, economical way to help the immune system maintain or regain its power against the countless antigens we face. Well, thanks to impressive scientific research and innovative manufacturing techniques, there is such an ingredient readily available over-the-counter. Beta-1,3-D-glucan (beta glucan) has demonstrated significant benefits for immune function.

Beta glucan is a simple polysaccharide (sugar/carbohydrate molecule) extracted from the cell wall of common baker's yeast. Although conventional medical scientists once dismissed beta glucan as nonsense because of its simplicity, it has now been confirmed that beta glucan profoundly and positively activates a powerful immune-system response.

While most of the scientific community resisted this discovery, a few pioneers proceeded and confirmed beta glucan's value.

A brief history

The story of beta glucan begins with the study of a drug used extensively in Europe, called Zymosan. This immune stimulator is made up of a crude mixture of yeast cell wall materials synthesized into a drug. Louis Pillemer, Ph.D., and his colleagues first studied the drug in the 1940s. It was during this research that Dr. Pillemer's group discovered that Zymosan, a combination of proteins, lipids, and polysaccharides, was able to nonspecifically modulate the immune system. This means it could activate the immune response regardless of the type of invader (i.e., virus, bacteria, or tumor).

In the 1960s, Nicholas DiLuzio, Ph.D., conducted additional research at Tulane University. It was Dr. DiLuzio's research that actually uncovered the active component of Zymosan. Beta-1,3-D-glucan was first identified as the immune-activating compound within the drug. From there, scientists tried to determine just how beta glucan worked.

In the 1980s, Joyce Czop, Ph.D., from Harvard University, unlocked the remaining mystery. Dr. Czop found specific receptor sites for beta glucan, specifically the 1,3 linkage of the cell, that matches a site on the surface of the macrophage. As we discussed in Chapter One, the macrophage is the first line of defense in our immune system; it plays a pivotal role in the activation of the entire immune response. Dr. Czop found that when beta glucan activates the macrophages, a myriad of immunological action and reaction occurs.

Although most of the research had been conducted via test tube (*in vitro*) or intravenously (IV), research in the late 1980s at Baylor College of Medicine confirmed the oral effectiveness of a purified beta glucan. This research, sponsored by the ImmuDyne Corporation, was important as it established the oral effectiveness of beta glucan and helped determine an adequate dose for the purified material. This is significant since it is much easier and more cost-effective to take something by mouth versus IV. Today, research continues on this innovative immune system activator.

Reviewing the research

Dr. Czop's work was a turning point in beta glucan research. By identifying the specific receptor on the macrophage that binds with beta glucan, we can more fully understand how this ingredient works and why it is so effective. From a scientific perspective, this is very important.

Dr. Czop discovered that the receptor site is a protein complex that appears to be present throughout the whole life cycle of the macrophage, even when it is first developed in the bone marrow. It has been confirmed that when the macrophage encounters the beta glucan molecule, the macrophage becomes activated. This triggers all the macrophage's powerful immune-stimulating capabilities. Remember, the macrophage serves many important functions, including the "eating" of antigens and cellular debris, and communicating with the T-cells to "tag" antigens in preparation for future attacks. In addition, the macrophage stimulates bone marrow production of immune-supporting substances.

In the 1970s, most of Dr. DiLuzio's research focused on using beta glucan as a complement to conventional therapies. His research successfully demonstrated beta glucan's effectiveness against hepatitis, leukemia, and wound-healing in animal models. Other researchers have confirmed the following:

O **Anti-infective.** By itself, beta glucan is a broad-spectrum, anti-infective agent that can eliminate bacteria, viruses, fungi, and parasites. When combined with an antibiotic, the macrophage stimulation of beta glucan can actually enhance the effectiveness of the drug.

O **Anti-cancer.** Numerous animal studies and anecdotal evidence has clearly shown beta glucan to be effective in treating many forms of cancer. When combined with anti-cancer treatments such as chemotherapy and radiation, beta glucan not only protects against the extensive adverse side effects of these treatments, it also enhances their effectiveness.

Let's hear what the scientific communit

"This demonstration of bactericidal enhancement via oral dosing suggests an application for beta-1,3-glucan as a component in a combined modality with conventional anti-infective agents. Beta glucan, through the stimulation of host defense systems, creates a more supportive environment within the body to assist the primary killing action of the conventional agent."

—Phil Wyde, Ph.D.

BAYLOR COLLEGE OF MEDICINE, HOUSTON, TX

"A cascade of interactions and reactions initiated by macrophage regulatory factors can be envisioned to occur and to eventuate in conversion of the glucan-treated host to an arsenal of defense...beta-1,3-glucan is at least 100 times more active than mannan (from aloe)."

—Joyce K. Czop, Ph.D.

DEPARTMENT OF RHEUMATOLOGY AND IMMUNOLOGY,
HARVARD MEDICAL SCHOOL

"Of all substances tested, glucan was the only substance to exhibit a particularly marked enhancement of the proliferative phase of wound healing. It appears, from these experiments, that the effect observed by others in terms of the activation of reticuloendothelial function by glucan and the activation of macrophages, both locally and systematically, also apply to activation of macrophages in healing wounds."

—S.J. Leibovich

THE WEIZMANN INSTITUTE OF SCIENCE,
REHOVOT, ISRAEL

is saying about beta glucan...

"Glucan was found to be an effective (substance) in inducing macrophage-mediated destruction in malignant lesions in animals and humans. Glucan has caused either complete or partial resolution of 100 percent of the human lesions into which it has been injected intralesionally."
—Peter Mansell, M.D.
McGILL UNIVERSITY CANCER RESEARCH UNIT,
VICTORIA HOSPITAL, MONTREAL, CANADA

"The broad spectrum of immunopharmacological activities of glucan includes not only the modification of certain bacterial, fungal, viral, and parasitic infection, but also inhibition of tumor growth."
—Nicholas DiLuzio, Ph.D.
DEPARTMENT OF PHYSIOLOGY,
TULANE UNIVERSITY SCHOOL OF MEDICINE

"Beta-1,3-glucan is a potent macrophage stimulant and is beneficial in the therapy of experimental bacterial, viral, and fungal diseases."
—William Browder, M.D.
DEPARTMENT OF SURGERY AND PHYSIOLOGY,
TULANE UNIVERSITY SCHOOL OF MEDICINE

"Glucan (beta-1,3) has been shown to enhance macrophage function dramatically, and to increase nonspecific host resistance to a variety of bacterial, viral, fungal, and parasitic infections."
—Myra L. Patchen, Ph.D.
DEPARTMENT OF EXPERIMENTAL HEMATOLOGY AND RADIATION SCIENCES,
ARMED FORCES RADIOLOGY RESEARCH INSTITUTE

○ **Topical agent.** Beta glucan is very effective as a wound healer. A combination of a topical antibiotic and beta glucan may prove to be extremely beneficial. We will learn more about the exciting area of skin applications of beta glucan later in this chapter.

The United States Armed Forces Radiobiology Institute conducted one of the most remarkable studies using oral beta glucan. In a well-controlled study, rats were given a lethal dose of radiation. Amazingly, 70 percent of the animals were completely protected from the effects when given a dose of yeast-derived beta glucan by mouth after the radiation.

Even the fishing industry has taken advantage of the benefits of beta glucan. In a 1994 article, *Modulators in Fish Immune Response*, the authors described how beta glucan was used in Atlantic salmon and catfish. The beta glucan increased the fish's resistance to a variety of bacterial pathogens.

Numerous other examples of the power of beta glucan exist in the scientific literature. Let's take a quick look:

○ **Melanoma.** Peter Mansell, M.D., of the McGill University Cancer Research Unit in Victoria Hospital in Montreal, Canada, injected beta glucan into subcutaneous nodules (i.e., lumps under the skin) of malignant melanoma. Subsequent biopsies of the injection sites found no evidence of the melanoma; just a collection of obviously activated macrophages.

○ **Skin ulcers.** One study involved women with recurrent malignant ulcers of the chest wall following mastectomy and radiation for breast cancer. Researchers found the ulcers completely healed after an application of beta glucan. Large pressure ulcers were also healed when the same material was used to treat a group of patients at the New Orleans Charity Hospital. The complete lack of infection and rapid growth of normal skin were additional, unexpected benefits.

○ **HIV.** The first human study on beta glucan's systemic effect (i.e., whole body rather than just one part) was done in the mid-1980s, featuring patients with advanced HIV (Human Immunodeficiency Virus) infection. Even in this case of severe immune system deficiency, the beta glucan increased immune system activity.

○ **Free-radical scavenger.** As an antioxidant, beta glucan is a powerful free-radical scavenger. Myra Patchen, Ph.D., found that beta glucan is able to protect blood macrophages from free radical attack during and after radiation, allowing these cells to continue their important immune functions. Free-radical-scavenging evaluations were repeated in different models to confirm the impressive antioxidant effect of beta glucan.

○ **Leukemia.** Several studies have shown beta glucan to be effective in the treatment of leukemia in animal models. These same studies also evaluated the combination of beta glucan with chemotherapy and/or radiation. Fifty-six percent of the animals were cured when combined therapy was used.

○ **Viral hepatitis.** Dr. DiLuzio and colleagues found beta glucan to be effective in animal studies on viral hepatitis. The researchers concluded that beta glucan treatment increased survival time, inhibited the progression of the disease, and stimulated the immune system.

○ **E. coli.** In 1990, researchers published their findings on E. coli bacteria in the *Scandinavian Journal of Immunology*. While the untreated animals died within 12 hours, the bacterial counts of the group treated with beta glucan measured zero after 24 hours.

The importance of vitamin C

Two-time Nobel Laureate Linus Pauling, Ph.D., showed conclusively that vitamin C stimulates the immune system and offers great protection against many illnesses. Dr. Pauling proved again that he was far ahead of his time. Today, many researchers finally agree that this simple vitamin packs a lot of power.

"Supplementation with vitamin C has been shown to help fight infections from virtually all pathogens," writes Dr. Pizzorno in his book, *Total Wellness*. "Even moderate levels of vitamin C supplementation in apparently healthy elderly adults on a supposedly adequate diet results in significant immune enhancement."

Recent research has shown that vitamin C and beta glucan form a perfect partnership. Researchers have discovered that macrophages utilize a large amount of vitamin C to accomplish their many responsibilities.

The vitamin C content in a macrophage cell can reach 40 times higher than the vitamin C content in the blood. In addition, macrophages activated with beta glucan exhibit a significant drop in their vitamin C content. Researchers believe this might lead to an exhaustion of their free-radical-scavenging capacity. It could also lead to impaired enzyme activity and movement within the macrophage. This is important, since it is the enzymes within the macrophage that actually "digest" the antigen.

Not only does vitamin C help the macrophage, the beta glucan has been shown to actually enhance the effectiveness of vitamin C. It's the ideal nutrient marriage.

Benefits to the skin

Not surprisingly, researchers are looking for other effective applications for this promising immune-stimulating natural ingredient. As it turns out, beta-glucan-containing products can provide incredible benefits to the skin.

Macrophages are present in all the organs of our body, including blood, liver, nervous system tissues, and skin. We used to think of our skin as merely an outer shield. Actually, our skin is the largest immune system organ of the human body.

The outer layer of the skin is called the epidermis. It contains up to five percent of the body's macrophages, known as Langerhans cells. Each of these macrophages in the epidermis has a body and long-reaching extensions. Because of these extensions, Langerhans cells literally form a fishnet within the upper layer of the skin, reaching most of the skin's cells.

The effect of a cosmetic regimen containing beta-1,3-D-glucan on the signs of aging in the skin was evaluated in 150 women, ages 35 to 60.

27% improvement in skin hydration

47% improvement in lines and wrinkles

60% increase in firmness and elasticity

26% skin color improvement

34% skin renewal

The role of Langerhans cells is extremely important. They carry out defensive and regulating functions within the skin. As with any macrophage, Langerhans cells are initially manufactured in the bone marrow. When they move from the bone marrow to the epidermis, they support the integrity of the skin.

The skin is constantly repairing itself. Its macrophages are responsible for cleaning and restoring damaged areas. As we age, the immune system's ability to respond to new challenges declines. The skin becomes less able to heal itself and cope with infection.

Beta glucan nourishes beauty as well as immune function. The cosmetic effect of products containing beta glucan was evaluated in 150 women, ages 35 to 60. Here are the results:

—A 27 percent improvement in skin hydration was observed after eight weeks of using the beta glucan regimen twice a day.

—There was a 47 percent improvement in lines and wrinkles at the end of the study.

—Firmness and elasticity increased by 60 percent, and skin color improved by 26 percent.

—Skin renewal was increased by 34 percent compared to the control group.

The cosmetic products (a serum and a cream) containing beta glucan at a concentration of 10 mg per ounce were applied after using an exfoliating toner containing salicylic acid. Using an exfoliator prior to applying beta glucan was important: It removed the superficial layer of dead skin, thereby exposing more Langerhans cell extensions to the beta glucan.

Unlike other skin care product ingredients, beta glucan is actively drawn into the Langerhans cells. Best of all, beta glucan is perfectly safe to use topically. It actually helps skin that has been damaged by other topical skin chemicals. In 1991, researchers observed the anti-irritant effect of beta glucan when it was used in combination with otherwise severe, irritation-causing levels of lactic acid. Beta glucan also has a synergistic effect with retinoic acid (Retin-A), another anti-aging topical. Similar to antibiotics, antifungals, and anti-cancer treatments, beta glucan can actually enhance the effectiveness of Retin-A.

Another factor to consider when dealing with the skin is ultraviolet (UV) light. Langerhans cells in the skin are very sensitive to environmental factors, including UV light. We know that UV light can suppress the immune system. In fact, UV light has been used to treat certain autoimmune skin diseases. Autoimmune conditions occur when the body's immune system attacks itself. (For more information on autoimmune conditions, refer to the question-and-answer section in Chapter Four.)

After even a brief exposure to UV light, the skin loses some Langerhans cells. This may explain at least partially how UV light undermines the immune system. When the first cell in the immune reaction chain is not in place, the rest of the immune system has trouble functioning. And, of course, this results in a higher rate of infections and tumors. We recommend the combination of a sunscreen and a beta-glucan-containing topical product.

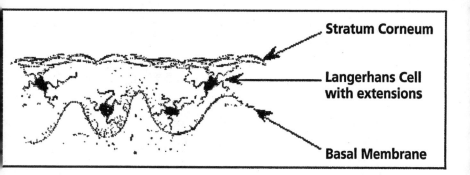

Stratum Corneum

Langerhans Cell
with extensions

Basal Membrane

Experiments with beta glucan indicate that it protects Langerhans cells after UV light exposure. In one study, a 0.05 percent external application of beta glucan prevented redness of the skin, skin cell damage, and depletion of Langerhans cells by more than 50 percent. Keep in mind, beta glucan does not act as a sunscreen. However, by protecting and stimulating the Langerhans cells, they become more resistant to damage. It also helps that beta glucan is such a powerful antioxidant and free-radical scavenger.

Not surprisingly, beta glucan also appears beneficial in cases of skin cancer, the most common type of human cancer. According to the American Cancer Society, more than 9,000 people in the United States died of skin cancer in 1995. Nearly all the 800,000-plus cases of basal and squamous cell skin cancer diagnosed each year in the United States are due to ultraviolet radiation from the sun. It only makes sense that beta glucan is a useful tool in cases of skin cancer prevention and treatment.

Beta glucan has further benefits topically. The wound-healing ability of beta glucan in general has been firmly established. One study compared several topical agents; only beta glucan showed any significant beneficial effect on actually healing the wound. The other over-the-counter and prescription products had no effect.

As the mass market catches up with the enthusiasm throughout the scientific community, we are sure to hear more about this powerful substance. Already, many major health magazines have recognized the benefits of beta glucan and the skin:

○ "...[beta glucan] may, in fact, be the first true anti-aging ingredient to go into moisturizers."
   —*Longevity*
○ "...a dynamic discovery that offers extraordinary benefits in whatever formulas include it."
   —*Let's Live*
○ "...an intriguing new 'youth' ingredient in skin boosting creams."
   —*Longevity*

○ "The visible result is skin with enhanced vitality, which is smoother and more supple."
   —*Muscle and Fitness*
○ "...patients experienced improvements in the quality and texture of their skin."
   —*Shape*
○ "[Beta glucan} seems to challenge the skin to correct whatever is wrong..."
   —*American Salon*

Summary

The incredible and far-reaching benefits of beta glucan have been researched for decades. Today, beta glucan is proving to be a highly effective natural ingredient for both oral and topical use.

When combined with vitamin C, beta glucan is even more effective as the activated macrophage relies heavily on vitamin C to carry out its important functions. Research has shown that replenishing vitamin C loss at the time when you introduce beta glucan provides optimum benefit. Based on the new understanding of macrophage activation, the combination of beta glucan and vitamin C is the most advanced, preferred physiological application.

Specific questions on toxicity, dosage, quality, and other important issues still remain. Join us in the next chapter for a conversation designed to get some answers to the remaining questions about beta glucan.

Chapter Four

A conversation with the expert

Let's set the scene for this next chapter. Take a moment to relax. Kick back in your favorite easy chair or settle on the couch. It's time to have a conversation with the expert. Imagine the three of us sitting together in your living room "chatting" about beta glucan. In this chapter, you will have the opportunity to put yourself in the seat of a research journalist talking with a research scientist. This format is designed to ensure you get all of your questions answered on this important topic.

Leonid Ber, M.D., received his doctorate in internal medicine from Yaroslavle State Medical Institute in Yaroslavle, Russia. Dr. Ber focused his attention on hematology, immunology, and intensive chemotherapy at the Central Hematological Institute in Moscow, Russia.

Karolyn A. Gazella is the president and founder of IMPAKT Communications, an innovative publishing company specializing in educational health information. She is the author of two books, several booklets, and has written hundreds of articles for consumers and professionals alike.

For convenience and readability, the questions are placed within three categories:
1. General
2. Safety/dosage/conditions
3. Quality
So, let's get started.

General

Karolyn A. Gazella: How did you first get involved with beta glucan?

Leonid Ber, M.D.: Actually, it was quite by accident. As a hematologist and an immunologist, I had patients with immune suppression from leukemia and other immune diseases. We used a drug called Zymosan, which is still a registered pharmaceutical drug in certain European countries, including Russia, where I was a practicing physician. Zymosan was used to boost bone marrow production in patients undergoing chemotherapy and radiation. This product, which is an injection, contains glucan, but it is not a purified form. Because of this, allergic reactions were quite common. Also because it is an injectable, there is a great deal of infection from the injection into the skin. When I heard about the research regarding a purified glucan, I was interested immediately. That led me to work with ImmuDyne, a company which focuses on glucan research. I was in charge of the research and development area that determined how to make glucan better and how it best can be used. Today, I am the Chief Operating Officer and on the board of directors.

KG: Why do you think this ingredient is so effective?

LB: It is a very simple ingredient. It almost sounds too simple to be effective. However, now that we have determined that these molecules have certain requirements in order to become active, we are discovering that it's not so simple. I think this particular ingredient is so effective in stimulating the immune system because it directly activates the macrophage, one of the most important components of the immune response. The fact that there is a receptor site on the macrophage that fits directly with beta glucan is very important. This tells us that the two are really meant for each other and that's how they can be so effective.

KG: Can beta glucan be used as a preventive?

LB: Yes. Individuals who want to keep their immune system healthy and strong can use a lower dosage of beta glucan as a powerful preventive. It is also ideal for those who are in good health but have a family history of immune-compromised conditions, such as cancer or diabetes. Many people use beta glucan to get through the cold and flu season, or if they are travelling on an airplane with 100 people sneezing and coughing. It does make the immune system stronger and more resistant.

KG: What conditions will benefit most from beta glucan therapy?

LB: Conditions that require a strong immune system, or any immune-compromised illness. Definitely people with cancer or tumors will benefit from beta glucan. Also, any type of chronic or acute infection will benefit. Because the macrophage activity is non-specific, it doesn't matter if the condition is bacterial, viral, or fungal. Beta glucan will help the condition. The macrophage simply determines if it belongs or doesn't belong—if it is yours or not yours. That's why beta glucan is so effective for so many conditions.

KG: What does the future hold for beta glucan?

LB: I definitely see this field growing, with new formulations and new synergies discovered. We may be able to use this ingredient in the form of ear drops, rectal applications, or more topical formulations. There is great healing potential. My hope is that as the oncology community becomes more open-minded, beta glucan should become a standard supplemental therapy for people undergoing chemotherapy and radiation. I also see it as an important option for reviving the effectiveness of antibiotics. It's not a secret anymore that many antibiotics don't work. Beta glucan can revive these antibiotics by giving them a second life. It's all a matter of education and understanding. That's where I see the progress of beta glucan—in giving the right information and exploring the possible applications. Just think of the positive impact this ingredient would have on our health care if it could lower the percentage of antibiotic resistance by just five percent. I think it has the potential to reduce it by half. I see that as an incredible contribution.

Safety/dosage/conditions

KG: Are there safety concerns regarding beta glucan?

LB: Beta glucan is completely safe and non-toxic. In the 1960s, there was a very crude beta glucan product on the market that did cause some side effects. It was even believed that this inferior product caused some people to develop lupus. However, in its purified form, and given the advanced technology available to us today, three decades later, we are able to get a very high quality extract that is safe to take. In fact, in animal studies, extremely large dosages were given with no toxicity. Keep in mind, however, that large quantities of the ingredient are not necessary.

KG: Are there any drug interactions that people should be aware of, or any drugs people should avoid while taking beta glucan?

LB: No. In fact, much research has shown that beta glucan actually enhances the effectiveness of many drugs, especially antibiotic, antifungal, and cholesterol-lowering drugs. While these drugs are very specific to the condition, they rely on an effective immune response to get the job done. That's why the beta glucan can actually make them work better and stronger. There are no known adverse effects with beta glucan and prescription or over-the-counter drugs.

KG: Combining natural substances with drugs seems to be a growing area of interest in scientific circles. Will we continue to see research on natural substances used in concert with pharmaceutical drugs?

LB: I see this as a growing trend. This is called complementary therapy. The natural substance protects the body but also enhances the particular drug. Studies have shown this to be the case with chemotherapy and radiation drugs, as well as with some natural substances used in conjunction with AZT and AIDS. We will see more of this research during the next decade.

KG: Will this ingredient be a problem for people who are allergic to yeast?

LB: No. Even though beta glucan is derived from baker's yeast, it is a pure isolate and does not actually contain any yeast proteins that would cause an allergic reaction. It is very important to reduce the amount of yeast protein to the lowest standard possible. Even for individuals who are not allergic, yeast protein can act as a sensitizer for the immune system, causing the person to possibly develop allergies to other things or provoke other immune responses. In one study involving individuals consuming nutritional yeast, there was a higher percentage of lupus, which is an autoimmune condition. The theory is that consumption of the yeast protein may somehow wake up the disease. That's why it is so important to buy the purest form of beta glucan possible. You don't want impurities and you don't want excess yeast proteins.

KG: How does this product work for those suffering with candidiasis, or yeast overgrowth problems?

LB: This product works very effectively for people with candidiasis. Remember, the product is not really yeast; it is a highly purified extract of the yeast cell wall. The finished molecule helps stimulate the immune system to look for the enemy—in this case, yeast overgrowth. For this condition, however, you need to use a lower dose of beta glucan. You don't want to overload the beta glucan receptors on the macrophage. Those same receptors are what the macrophage uses to attack the invading fungal cells. That's why anti-fungal applications with beta glucan are more dose sensitive. There is a balance that needs to be maintained. You want to stimulate the immune cells, but not overload them so the receptor sites can remain unoccupied, active, and ready to attack. When beta glucan is used appropriately, it can be extremely effective for people suffering from candidiasis.

KG: Many people wonder if beta glucan can actually cause an over-stimulation of the immune system or lead to the development of an autoimmune condition?

LB: Beta glucan is a case where more is not necessarily better. People should always use beta glucan products as directed and buy the purest form of beta glucan possible. Unfortunately, some products on the market offer a form of beta glucan that contains very high dosages of yeast proteins. Taking these products is not advised. Extremely high dosages of beta glucan could actually shut down macrophage activity or deplete the body of vitamin C, since macrophages utilize large amounts of vitamin C. However, as long as the proper dosage of a purified standardized product is used for the proper condition, beta glucan is extremely safe and effective.

KG: How does beta glucan work for people suffering from autoimmune conditions such as rheumatoid arthritis, lupus, and others?

LB: Autoimmune diseases occur when the body attacks its own cells with specific immune system antibodies. These antibodies are produced by B-cells. Beta glucan does not affect these antibody-producing lymphocyte cells because they simply don't have the type of receptors that the macrophages have. Beta glucan is really the safest immune stimulant you can take if you have an autoimmune disorder. Another reason to consider beta glucan for an autoimmune situation is that these conditions are usually treated with immunosuppressive drugs and hormones. The purpose of this type of therapy is to reduce antibody production; however, other components of the immune-system response are suppressed as well. For example, prednisone (or other corticosteroid hormone drugs) suppress macrophage activity, which can lead to further immune system problems. Common complications of these drugs include fungal and other infections. Beta glucan has been shown to reduce the side effects of the medication without interfering with its treatment purpose.

KG: Why is the beta glucan so effective on so many different types of cancer?

LB: Cancer is a very complex disease. The better the cancer cell can masquerade to look like a normal cell, the less chance the immune system and the macrophages will have to recognize it and attack. These cancers, which are referred to as cancers with low immunogenecity (i.e., detecting an immune response), are the hardest to treat with either conventional or alternative methods. Beta glucan can take the "mask" off the cancer cells as it activates the macrophage's ability to recognize them as abnormal. This complements and improves the results of the anti-cancer program. Beta glucan is also effective against cancer because it works so well with conventional cancer drugs such as chemotherapy and radiation.

KG: What is the recommended dosage when using beta glucan as a preventive? For this purpose, is additional vitamin C needed?

LB: First of all, it is very important that beta glucan be taken on an empty stomach. This will enhance the effectiveness of the product, because the beta glucan passes through the stomach to the upper intestines. If the product is taken with food, it may pass through the system with the food and might not be exposed. Regarding dosages, as a preventive, I recommend 2.5 mg daily taken 30 minutes before a meal or two hours after a meal. Extra vitamin C is not necessary in these cases. The amount of vitamin C in a good multi-vitamin/mineral supplement will be adequate.

KG: What dosage do you recommend for people using beta glucan for an infection or specific immune-compromised conditions such as cancer?

LB: Obviously, these people require a stronger dose. I recommend 7.5 mg daily, sometimes even higher. I also recommend at least 400 mg of non-acidic vitamin C taken with the beta glucan. This will help reduce the chances of vitamin C deficiency, as well as enhance the effectiveness of the activated macrophages. Again, this should be taken on an empty stomach for optimum effectiveness. It is also important to remind people that it is safe to take beta glucan at this dosage in conjunction with chemotherapy, radiation, antibiotic antifungal, or cholesterol-lowering drugs. As I have explained, the beta glucan will actually enhance the effectiveness of these drugs. These individuals may be tempted to take even higher dosages of the beta glucan, thinking that more is better. This is not the case with beta glucan. We have found the optimum dosage for these individuals, and that is 7.5 mg daily with 400 mg of vitamin C.

KG: Although beta glucan has to be taken on an empty stomach, can it be taken with other supplements at the same time?

LB: Yes, with the exception of fiber supplements. It is the fiber in foods and supplements that the beta glucan can attach to and then be eliminated without macrophage receptors ever being exposed to it. For this reason, individuals should avoid taking beta glucan with food and fiber supplements. It can be taken with other nutritional supplements.

Quality

KG: How does beta glucan from the yeast cell wall compare to other sources of beta glucan, such as barley or mushrooms?

LB: Beta glucan from barley, oats, or other grains has been shown to have different composition and be impractical to use for specific immunological activation of the macrophages. The activity of beta glucan from mushrooms also varies, depending on the attributes of the actual active molecule. These other sources of beta glucan might have small portions of the important 1,3 molecule. Only beta glucan from the cell wall of baker's yeast has been shown to actually have a direct effect on the specific receptor site.

KG: Could you explain a little about the extraction process?

LB: The goal is to extract the molecule that has been shown in clinical studies to match the receptor site on the macrophage. For example, there is a beta-1,3-D-glucan molecule available in algae, but it does not have the activity. It does not fit into the macrophage receptor site to activate the immune system response. The proper molecule is beta 1,3-D-glucan from the yeast cell wall. We know precisely what the molecule is supposed to look like, so we extract that exact molecule. It is the skeleton of the yeast cell, with a backbone and branches. Each of the branches forms a spiral configuration and the entire molecule forms a triple helix. So, you see, it is a very specific molecule that has the immune-stimulating activity.

KG: I know there are 1,4 and 1,6 beta glucans available. How do they compare to the 1,3? What is the significance of the numbers 1,3?

LB: The 1,3 is the specific linkage within the molecule that is recognized by the macrophage receptor. It just so happens that 1,3 is what makes the specific key fit into the lock, so to speak. The 1,4 and 1,6 are totally different linkages that form totally different molecules with completely different properties. The research has shown that the 1,3 linkage has the effectiveness. If you use a molecule with 1,3, 1,4, and 1,6 beta glucans, chances are you will get an immune response. Once you take out the 1,3, you will not have the activity and you won't get an effective immune response. While the 1,4 and 1,6 still may work with the 1,3, it is not as pure and it won't be nearly as effective because they are totally different molecules. These molecules are soluble, whereas the 1,3 is insoluble. For an oral or topical application, the insoluble molecule has been shown to be the most potent and most therapeutic.

KG: How do you evaluate potency and effectiveness of a purified beta glucan product?

LB: A standard of purity and effectiveness has been established. Obviously, the best beta glucan to purchase is the pure beta 1,3. This beta glucan will provide you with the most power at the lowest dosage.

KG: How can individuals determine if they are getting a high-quality beta glucan product?

LB: There is a trademark symbol that guarantees the potency and quality of a standardized, purified beta glucan product. Look for the symbol YB13G. This symbol is designed to let consumers know that the product has been standardized for potency and that it is pure and protein-free. This symbol also lets you know that the product contains insoluble 1,3 beta glucan with the triple helix configuration. This is very important in terms of effectiveness. Because there are a lot of different sources of beta glucan, this symbol also lets you know that you are purchasing beta glucan from the yeast cell wall, which is also important in terms of insolubility and effectiveness. Also, purchase your beta glucan product from a reputable company that has a history of working with beta glucan.

Summary

As with any substance you put into your body, beta glucan should be used with care. Although this substance is completely safe in its purified, standardized form, taking more is not necessarily better. It is critical to use the dosages Dr. Ber and other researchers recommend. These dosages are based on solid scientific evidence gleaned from several decades of research studies.

Choosing the highest quality beta glucan product may become more challenging as manufacturers jump on the beta glucan bandwagon. Stick with reliable manufacturers who are used to dealing with beta glucan products. Look for the YB13G symbol on the label; this is your indication that the product matches the effective, purified form used in the studies. The YB13G product meets high standards of purity, potency, insolubility, and has the important three-dimensional configuration.

Once you find a beta glucan product you are comfortable with, the rest is up to you. When added to a comprehensive immune-system activation plan, beta glucan can provide powerful benefits. But remember, there is no such thing as a cure-all, especially when we are dealing with the complex immune system. Even beta glucan can't do it alone. It needs your help and the support of a truly well-rounded, health-promoting strategy.

Chapter Five

Closing comments

Science has provided a fascinating glimpse at the most powerful health-promoting system known—the immune system. The workings of this internal army are nothing short of spectacular. In almost magical fashion, trillions of cells patrol around the clock to keep us healthy. They are ready to fight for us, and if we support them properly, they will win!

Unfortunately, the immune army inside often fails to conquer its enemy, as evidenced by the growing rate of cancer in our country. Decades ago, then-President Richard Nixon declared a "war on cancer." Today, we are no closer to a cure as researchers pine for a magic bullet.

As reported in Dr. Quillin's comprehensive book, *Beating Cancer with Nutrition*, former president of Stanford University, Donald Kennedy, called the war on cancer "a medical Vietnam." Dr. Linus Pauling referred to it as "largely a fraud." And John Bailar, M.D., Ph.D., former editor of the *Journal of the National Cancer Institute*, concluded that the war on cancer is "a qualified failure."

"Grouped together, the average cancer patient has a 50/50 chance of living another five years, which are the same odds he/she had in 1971," reports Dr. Quillin. "Newly diagnosed cancer incidence continues to escalate..."

While new anti-cancer drugs continue to enter the market, only time will tell if they will make a dent in cancer's unyielding armor. The most recent discovery cuts off the blood supply to solid tumors in hopes they will stop growing and/or even die. While this is believed to be the biggest breakthrough in anti-cancer medicine for decades, it will take years to fine-tune this therapy. In addition, this new therapy does not work on all cancers.

And cancer is not the only villain. New immune system challenges include the AIDS epidemic, the ineffectiveness of antibiotics, the ever-increasing amount of environmental toxins, and the incredible rise in preservatives and hormones in our food supply. We desperately need immune system support.

There is no such thing as a magic cure-all. We believe a comprehensive approach is the only successful approach. Combined with other factors such as diet, lifestyle, and attitude, beta glucan can serve as a phenomenal immune system activator.

Dr. Ber and I each have a personal connection with beta glucan and the immune system. Following are our individual final thoughts on this important topic.

Final thoughts from Dr. Ber

As a medical doctor trained as an immunologist, I am intricately aware of the power of the immune system. I have been fascinated by this power and have studied it extensively over the years. The human immune system has an incredible ability to heal.

Also during my medical career, I have witnessed first-hand the devastation that a weakened immune system can cause. I have seen the suffering connected with cancer and other immune-compromised conditions. The toll these conditions take on the health of this world is immense and at times incomprehensible.

When I learned that a sister of my friend, DJ, was diagnosed with cancer, I wanted to help. After the initial shock went away, we worked together to develop a plan for her. Beta glucan was a key player.

DJ's sister was 55 years old when she noticed she had trouble swallowing. It was discovered that a large tumor mass was almost completely obstructing her larynx and esophagus. Her doctor gave her no more than 30 days to live, unless she started radiation, which she refused. DJ was already giving her various vitamins and minerals that didn't seem to do anything to the tumor. A portion of the tumor was ulcerated and easily accessible, so we decided to split the dose of beta glucan between an oral supplement she took daily with water, and a local application, where she would suspend beta glucan in flaxseed oil to keep the beta glucan in the area of the tumor.

After a month of her doing this regimen religiously, an X-ray revealed the tumor had shrunk. Her oncologist's comment was, "I told you the radiation would help." He was speechless when DJ responded, "She is not on radiation."

Another month passed and DJ called me in a panic, "My sister's tumor is in the toilet!" The body had rejected the tumor and the portion of the esophagus that it had affected was healing quickly. A local biopsy did not reveal any tumor cells. Everybody felt relieved.

Unfortunately, several months later, we discovered that DJ's sister's cancer had already metastasized. While the original location still did not show any sign of recurrence of tumor, the spreading cancer got the best of her. However, even though DJ's sister died of cancer, it was incredible to see the healing power of this natural substance known as beta glucan.

I get dozens of calls from doctors every day. Beta glucan is clearly becoming recognized as a valuable tool in their natural arsenal.

It has always been my dream to make a difference, to help stop the suffering, to make an impact on my profession, and to leave a legacy of innovative scientific discovery and compassion.

I believe beta glucan can have such a profound, far-reaching effect on the health of this nation. Someday, beta glucan will be acknowledged as one of the most significant discoveries of our time.

Final thoughts from Karolyn

Sometimes when I talk in front of a group or I'm interviewed for a radio program, I feel slightly fragmented. I am really three different people offering three different perspectives. First, as the owner of a publishing company, I can discuss topics that relate to publishing or running a business. Secondly, as a research journalist, I need to convey details to my readers or listeners in an understandable, accurate, and relevant way. Finally, and most importantly, I am a healthcare consumer, someone who has fought serious illness and won!

In the summer of 1994, my only sister (who was also my second employee) was diagnosed with breast cancer. Then, five months later, my mom (who was my first employee) died of advanced pancreatic cancer. Less than three months after my mom died—two days after my 33rd birthday—I was operated on for ovarian cancer. Three cancers within eight months!

The horror of my mom's cancer was unbelievable. The cancer ripped through her body quickly and uncontrollably. Just a week before she became very sick, she was in the warehouse shipping boxes of magazines. I brought her to the hospital for what we thought would be gallbladder surgery. Three weeks later, Mom was dead. The cancer had moved swiftly from her pancreas, to her bile duct, and throughout her internal organs. At the time of her diagnosis, she had five different tumors in her liver alone.

She died during the Christmas holiday season. That seemed appropriate for Mom, because she was such a spiritual person. It was her strength that helped me overcome my cancer. Today, I rely on her spiritual influence to keep me healthy.

However, both my sister Kathi and I realized right away that it would take more than Mom's strong spirit to keep us healthy. She couldn't do the job alone! We made important lifestyle changes and utilized an aggressive nutritional supplement program to help us overcome our cancers. Today, we are both in great health.

I rely on a beta glucan product to boost my immune system. My first experience with beta glucan was during the early stages of a miserable cold. I took a potent beta glucan product and within 24 hours, I had kicked the cold from my system. As I began researching the product more thoroughly, I recommended it to several people. The success story I am most thankful for involves my dearest friend's dad.

Jerry is a hard-working farmer living in rural Wisconsin. At age 65, he could work harder than a man half his age. Then Jerry and his family received some devastating news: He had prostate cancer that had spread outside the prostate. Faced with many difficult decisions, Jerry decided to try a new procedure in which they insert nearly 100 different radiation-filled bee bees into the area with the cancer.

Unfortunately, Jerry and his family were not informed of the many side effects that could accompany this therapy. We tried everything to alleviate his pain and discomfort, to no avail. He was unable to work. The conventional medical doctors who did the procedure pretty much turned their backs on him. They were unable to provide him with any relief.

Fortunately, Jerry is a patient man. He was willing to try different alternative therapies until we were able to find something that worked for him. On Easter Sunday, 1998, I gave Jerry a bottle of the most potent beta glucan product available—7.5 mg with vitamin C added—and instructed him to take one capsule every day on an empty stomach. After being on the beta glucan/vitamin C therapy for only a few days, he felt considerably better. After only one week, Jerry was comfortably sitting on his tractor, working his farm fields. Today, at age 70, he's that same hard-working farmer! While we are not sure if the cancer is gone completely, his prognosis looks very good.

What made this product perfect for Jerry was that he only had to take one capsule daily and it didn't upset his stomach. With a history of digestive problems, Jerry was unable to tolerate many of the other nutritional supplements I had recommended. In addition, the beta glucan has been scientifically proven to enhance the effectiveness of radiation. I think the beta glucan was able to strengthen Jerry's immune system and actually improve the effectiveness of the radioactive bee bees.

This is just one of the many success stories I have heard about beta glucan. These stories and my own personal experience have certainly made a believer out of me. We have not heard the last of this incredible ingredient.

I know how it feels to be overcome with a serious, life-threatening illness. It's almost as if your own immune system stops working, leaving you to fend for yourself against your internal enemy. However, never lose sight that the power of your immune system can almost always be activated.

There's no better feeling than when you conquer an illness. Think of how much better you feel after having the flu for a few days. You're just so happy to be feeling better that your mood picks up and you're more appreciative of your good health than ever before. I, too, know that feeling.

I live my life differently now. I do a variety of things to give my immune system the upper hand. I have experienced the power of my own immune system. And you can, too!

Summary

We have written this book in an effort to help you recognize—and unleash—the incredible power of your immune system. Armed with the right information, you can gain optimum health by effectively preventing and treating serious, immune-compromised conditions. Clearly, the more people who know about beta glucan, the more people will be helped by this powerful immune-system activator.

Reviewing the highlights

We've packed a lot of information into this book. For your convenience, here is a review of the highlights.

○ **Immune system**—The immune system is made up of a complex mixture of cells, fluids, and organs working together to keep us healthy. Around the clock, the trillions of specialized immune system cells team up to protect us from illness. There are 54 billion white blood cells alone circulating and patrolling.

○ **Macrophage**—The macrophage cells are very important components of the immune system. These large cells circulate throughout the body "eating" viruses, bacteria, and a host of other toxins. The macrophage also activates the immune response by causing a chain reaction with other cells. Furthermore, macrophages "tag" dead antigens (i.e., viruses, fungi, and parasites) so the immune system can recognize them the next time they enter the body. Macrophages are extensively involved in everyday elimination of toxins, maintenance of intestinal flora, protection from infection and tumor, and overall health.

○ **Toxic environment**—The task of our immune system is made even more challenging as we battle an increasing number of external toxins in the air we breathe, the foods we eat, and the water we drink. Pesticides, preservatives, antibiotics in the food supply, cancer-causing substances in the air—these are just a few examples of toxins that negatively influence the immune system.

○ **Weakened immune system**—There are countless examples that illustrate the link between a weak immune system and the development of disease. The most common is cancer. Other examples include HIV/AIDS, candidiasis, diabetes, and diseases associated with aging.

○ **Immune system support**—There are many steps we can take to stimulate a positive immune-system response. A comprehensive immune-system strategy should include a healthful diet, positive immune-activating lifestyle choices (i.e., no smoking, regular exercise), a positive attitude, and nutritional supplements. Many natural substances are available to support the health of the immune system. (For more information, refer to Appendix II.)

○ **Beta glucan**—Science has discovered the benefits of a purified, standardized extract of the yeast cell wall known as beta-1,3-D-glucan. When taken orally, as a nutritional supplement, this ingredient can actually activate macrophage activity and provide incredible support to the immune system. This ingredient is completely safe. In fact, when combined with many prescription and over-the-counter drugs, it will enhance the effectiveness of the drug, while protecting the body from its side effects. It is vital that the product purchased is a standardized, purified form of beta glucan that is the 1,3 component of the molecule. Quality can vary from product to product. Look for the YB13G logo. Also, remember to take the product as directed. More is not necessarily better. With the higher dosage of 7.5 mg, it is best to combine vitamin C. For optimum benefit, beta glucan should be taken on an empty stomach.

References

1. Enhanced healing of decubitus ulcers by topical application of particulate glucan. Tulane University School of Medicine Research Summary:1984.(Abstract)

2. The acute oral toxicity study of beta-1,3-glucan in rats. Essex testing Clinic, Report: 1990.

3. Anti-free radical activity of beta-1,3-glucan molecule. Seporga Laboratories, Sophia Antipolis, France Research report:1990.

4. Beta,3-glucan: effect of oral application on interleukinl-1 release in mice. Baylor College of Medicine, Research Report 1994.

5. Abel, G. and Czop, J.K. Stimulation of human monocyte beta-glucan receptors by glucan particles induces production of TNF-alpha and IL-1 beta. *Int. J. Immunopharmacol.* 14:1363-1373, 1992.

6. Almdahl, S.M., Bogwald, J., Hoffman, J., Sjunneskog, C. and Seljelid, R. The effect of splenectomy on Escherichia coli sepsis and its treatment with semisoluble aminated glucan. *Scand. J. Gastroenterol.* 22:261-267, 1987.

7. Babineau, T.J., Marcello, P., Swails, W., Kenler, A., Bistrian, B. and Forse, R.A. Randomized phase I/II trial of a macrophage-specific immunomodulator (PGG-glucan) in high-risk surgical patients. *Ann. Surg.* 220:601-609, 1994.

8. Ber, L., Yeast-derived beta-1,3-D-glucan: An adjuvant concept, *The American Journal of Natural Medicine*, 4(9):21-25, Nov. 1997.

9. Ber, L., Beta-1,3-D-glucan: The skin connection, *Nature's Impact*, Dec./Jan. 1998.

10. Block, M.A., Ear infections & bacterial resistance, *Nature's Impact* magazine, February/March 1998.

11. Bogwald, J., Johnson, E. and Seljelid, R. The cytotoxic effect of mouse macrophages stimulated in vitro by a beta-1,3-D-glucan from yeast cell walls. *Scand. J. Immunol.* 15:297-304, 1982.

12. Bowers, G.J., Patchen, M.L., MacVittie, T.J., Hirsch, E.F. and Fink, M.P. Glucan enhances survival in an intra-abdominal infection model. *J. Surg. Res.* 47:183-188, 1989.

13. Browder, I.W., Sherwood, E., Williams, D., Jones, E., McNamee, R. and DiLuzio, N. Protective effect of glucan-enhanced macrophage function in experimental pancreatitis. *Am. J. Surg.* 153:25-33, 1987

14. Browder, I.W., Williams, D.L., Kitahama, A. and Di Luzio, N.R. Modification of post-operative C. albicans sepsis by glucan immunostimulation. *Int. J. Immunopharmacol.* 6:19-26, 1984.

15. Browder, W., Williams, D., Lucore, P., Pretus, H., Jones, E. and McNamee, R. Effect of enhanced macrophage function on early wound healing. *Surgery* 104:224-230, 1988.

16. Browder, W., Williams, D., Pretus, H., Olivero, G., Enrichens, F., Mao, P. and Franchello, A. Beneficial effect of enhanced macrophage function in the trauma patient. *Ann. Surg.* 211:605-12, discuss, 1990.

17. Browder, W., Williams, D., Pretus, H., Olivero, G., Enrichens, F. Mao, P. and Franchello, A. Beneficial Effect of Enhanced Macrophage Function in the Trauma Patients. *Ann. Surg* 211:605-613, 1990.

18. Browder, W., Williams, D., Sherwood, E., McNamee, R., Jones, E and DiLuzio, N. Synergistic effect of nonspecific immunostimulation and antibiotics in experimental peritonitis. *Surgery* 102:206-214, 1987.

19. Cassone, A., Bistoni, F., Cenci, E., Pesce, C.D., Tissi, L. and Marconi, P. Immunopotentiation of anticancer chemotherapy by Candida albicans, other yeasts and insoluble glucan in an experimental lymphoma model. *Sabouraudia.* 20:115-125, 1982.

20. Chorvatovicova, D. and Navarova, J. Suppressing effects of glucan on micronuclei induced by cyclophosphamide in mice. *Mutat. Res.* 282:147-150,1992.

21. Compton, R., Williams, D. and Browder, W. The beneficial effect of enhanced macrophage function on the healing of bowel anastomoses. *Am. Surg.* 62:14-18, 1996.

22. Cook, J.A., Holbrook, T.W. and Dougherty, W.J. Protective effect of glucan against visceral leishmaniasis in hamsters. *Infect. Immun.* 37:1261-1269, 1982.

23. Czop, J.K. and Austen, K.F. A beta-glucan inhibitable receptor on human monocytes: its identity with the phagocytic receptor for particulate activators of the alternative complement pathway. *J Immunol.* 134:2588-2593, 1985.

24. Czop, J.K., Gurish, M.F. and Kadish, J.L. Production and isolation of rabbit anti-idiotypic antibodies directed against the human monocyte receptor for yeast beta-glucans. *J. Immunol.* 145:995-1001, 1990.

25. Czop, J.K. and Kay, J. Isolation and characterization of beta-glucan receptors on human mononuclear phagocytes. *J. Exp. Med.* 173:1511-1520, 1991.

26. Di Luzio, N.R., Macrophage functional status and Neoplasia. Pathophysiology of the Reticuloendothelial System Altura BM, Saba. 1996.

27. Di Luzio, N.R., McNamee, R.B., Williams, D.L., Gilbert, K.M. and Spanjers, M.A., Glucan induced inhibition of tumor growth and enhancement of survival in a variety of transplantable and spontaneous murine tumor models. *Adv. Exp. Med. Biol.* 121A:269-290, 1980.

28. Di Luzio, N.R. and Williams, D.L. Protective effect of glucan against systemic Staphylococcus aureus septicemia in normal and leukemic mice. *Infect. Immun.* 20:804-810, 1978.

29. Di Renzo, L., Yefenof, E. and Klein, E. The function of human NK cells is enhanced by beta-glucan, a ligand of CR3 (CD11b/CD18). *Eur. J. Immunol.* 21:1755-1758, 1991.

30. DiLuzio, N.R. Immunopharmacology of glucan: a broad spectrum enhancer of host defense mechanism. *Trends in Pharmacological Sciences* 4:344-347, 1983.

31. Ferencik, M., Kotulova, D., Masler, L., Bergendi, L., Sandula, J. and Stefanovic, J. Modulatory effect of glucans on the functional and biochemical activities of guinea-pig macrophages. Methods Find.Exp. Clin. Pharmacol. 8:163-166, 1986.

32. Gazella, K. A., Homocysteine - Discovering the truth about heart disease, *Nature's Impact* magazine, June/July 1998.

33. Gazella, K.A., *The Thymus: Master Gland of Immunity*, IMPAKT Communications, Inc., Green Bay, 1996.

34. Gazella, K.A., *Buyer Be Wise! The Consumer's Guide to Buying Quality Nutritional Supplements*, IMPAKT Communications, Inc., Green Bay, 1998.

35. Fukase, S., Inoue, T., Arai, S. and Sendo, F. Tumor cytotoxicity of polymorphonuclear leukocytes in beige mice: linkage of high responsiveness to linear beta-1,3-D-glucan with the beige gene. *Cancer Res.* 47:4842-4847,1987.

36. Glovsky, M.M., Cortes-Haendchen, L., Ghekiere, L., Alenty, A., Williams, D.L. and Di Luzio, R. Effects of particulate beta-1,3 glucan on human, rat, and guinea pig complement activity. *J. Reticuloendothel. Soc.* 33:401-413, 1983.

37. Goldman, R. Characteristics of the beta-glucan receptor of murine macrophages. *Exp. Cell Res.* 174:481-490, 1988.

38. Hoffman, O.A., Olson, E.J. and Limper, A.H. Fungal beta-glucans modulate macrophage release of tumor necrosis factor-alpha in response to bacterial lipopolysaccharide. *Immunol. Lett.* 37:19-25, 1993.

39. Janusz, M.J., Austen, K.F. and Czop, J.K. Lysosomal enzyme release from human monocytes by particulate activators is mediated by beta-glucan inhibitable receptors. *J. Immunol.* 138:3897-3901, 1987.

40. Janusz, M.J., Austen, K.F. and Czop, J.K. Phagocytosis of heat-killed blastophores of Candida albicans by human monocytes beta-glucan receptors. *Immunology* 65:181-185, 1988.

41. Janusz, M.J., Austen, K.F. and Czop, J.K. Isolation of a yeast heptaglucoside that inhibits monocyte phagocytosis of zymosan particles. *J. Immunol.* 142:959-965, 1989.

42. Kanai, K., Kondo, E., Jacques, P.J. and Chihara, G. Immunopotentiating effect of fungal glucans as revealed by frequency limitation of postchemotherapy relapse in experimental mouse tuberculosis. *Jpn. J. Med. Sci. Biol.* 33:283-293, 1980.

43. Kenyon, A.J. Delayed wound healing in mice associated with viral alteration of macrophages. *Am. J. Vet. Res.* 44:652-656, 1983.

44. Kimura, A., Sherwood, R.L. and Goldstein, E. Glucan alteration of pulmonary antibacterial defense. *J. Reticuloendothel. Soc.* 34:1-11, 1983.

45. Kohut, M.L. and Davis, J.M. Effect of exercise on macrophage antiviral function in the lung. *J. of Am. College of Sports Medicine* 26:33, 1994.

46. Kunimoto, T., Baba, H. and Nitta, K. Antitumor polysaccharide-induced tumor-regressing factor in the serum of tumor-bearing mice: purification and characterization. *J. Biol. Response. Mod.* 5:225-235, 1986.

47. Lahnborg, G., Hedstrom, K.G and Nord, C.E. The effect of glucan - a host resistance activator - and ampicillin on experimental intra-abdominal sepsis. *J. of Reticuloendothelial Soc.* 32:347-353, 1982.

48. Lahnborg, G., Hedstrom, K.G. and Nord, C.E. Glucan-induced enhancement of host resistance in experimental intra-abdominal sepsis. *Eur. Surg. Res.* 14:401-408, 1982.

49. Lang, C.H. and Dobrescu, C. Interleukin-1 induces increases in glucose utilization are insulin mediated. *Life Sciences* 45:2127-2134, 1989.

50. Leibovich, S.J. and Danon, D. Promotion of Wound Repair in Mice by Application of Glucan. *J. of Reticuloendothelial Soc.* 27:1, 1978.

51. Mansell, P.W.A., Ichinose, H., Reed, R.J., Krementz, E.T., McNamee, R. and DiLuzio, N.R. Macrophage-mediated destruction of human malignant cells in vivo. *J. of the National Cancer Institute* 54, No.3:571, 1975.

52. Mansell, P.W.A., Rowden, G. and Hammer, C. Clinical Experiences with the Use of Glucan. In: Immune modulation and control of neoplasia by adjuvant therapy, New York: Raven Press, 1978,

53. Michaud, E., Feinstein, A., *Fighting Disease! The Complete Guide to Natural Immune Power*, Rodale Press, Inc., Pennsylvania, 1989.

54. Morikawa, K., Kikuchi, Y., Abe, S., Yamazaki, M. and Mizuno, D. Early cellular responses in the peritoneal cavity of mice to antitumor immunomodulators. *Gann.* 75:370-378, 1984.

55. Nicoletti, A., Nicoletti, G., Ferraro, G., Palmieri, G., Mattaboni, P. and Germogli, R. Preliminary evaluation of immunoadjuvant activity of an orally administered glucan extracted from Candida albicans. *Arzneimittelforschung.* 42:1246-1250, 1992.

56. Patchen, M.L. Radioprotectibe effect of oral administration of beta-1,3-glucan. Armed Forces Radiobiology Institute Bethesda, MD Research report:1989.(Abstract)

57. Patchen, M.L., Brook, I., Elliott, T.B. and Jackson, W.E. Adverse effects of pefloxacin in irradiated C3H/HeN mice: correction with glucantherapy. *Antimicrob. Agents Chemother.* 37:1882-1889, 1993.

58. Patchen, M.L., D'Alesandro, M.M., Brook, I., Blakely, W.F. and MacVittie, T.J. Glucan: Mechanisms Involved in Its "Radioprotective" Effect. *J. of Leukocyte Biology* 42:95-105, 1987.

59. Patchen, M.L. and MacVittie, T.J. Dose-dependent responses of murine pluripotent stem cells and myeloid and erythroid progenitor cells following administration of the immunomodulating agent glucan. *Immunopharmacology* 5:303-313, 1983.

60. Patchen, M.L. and MacVittie, T.J. Temporal response of murine pluripotent stem cells and myeloid progenitor cells to low-dose glucan treatment. *Acta Haemat.* 70:281-288, 1983.

61. Patchen, M.L. and MacVittie, T.J. Stimulated hemopoiesis and enhanced survival following glucan treatment in sublethally and lethally irradiated mice. *Int. J. Immunopharmacol.* 7:923-932, 1985.

62. Patchen, M.L. and MacVittie, T.J. Stimulated hemopoiesis and enhanced survival following glucan treatment in sublethally and lethally irradiated mice. *Int. J. Immunopharmac.* 6:923-932, 1985.

63. Patchen, M.L., MacVittie, T.J. and Jackson, W.E. Postirradiation glucan administration enhances the radioprotective effects of WR-2721. *Radiat. Res.* 117:59-69, 1989.

64. Patchen, M.L., MacVittie, T.J., Solberg, B.D. and Souza, L.M. Survival enhancement and hemopoietic regeneration following radiation exposure: therapeutic approach using glucan and granulocyte colony-stimulating factor. *Exp. Hematol.* 18:1042-1048, 1990.

65. Patchen, M.L., MacVittie, T.J. and Wathen, L.M. Effects of pre- and post-irradiation glucan treatment on pluripotent stem cells, granulocyte, macrophage and erythroid progenitor cells, and hemopoietic stromal cells. *Experientia.* 40:1240-1244, 1984.

66. Pizzorno, J., *Total Wellness*, Prima Publishing, California, 1998.

67. Pretus, H.A., Browder, I.W., Lucore, P., McNamee, R.B., Jones, E.L. and Williams, D.L. Macrophage activation decreases macrophage prostaglandin E2 release in experimental trauma. *J. Trauma.* 29:1152-6; discussion, 1989.

68. Proctor, J.W., Stiteler, R.D., Yamamura, Y., Mansell, P.W. and Winters, R. Effect of glucan and other adjuvants on the clearance of radiolabeled tumor cells from mouse lungs. *Cancer Treat. Rep.* 62:1873-1880, 1978.

69. Proctor, J.W., Yamamura, Y., DiLuzio, N.R., Mansell, P.W. and Harnaha, J., Development of a bioassay for the antitumor activity of biological response modifiers of the reticuloendothelial stimulant class, correlation with the outgrowth of lung tumor nodules. *Cancer Immunol. Immunother.* 10:197-202, 1981.

70. Quillin, P., Quillin, N., *Beating Cancer with Nutrition*, Revised Edition, Nutrition Times Press, Inc., Oklahoma, 1998.

71. Rasmussen Busund, L.T., Konopski, Z., Oian, P. and Seljelid, R. Killing of Escherichia coli by mononuclear phagocytes and neutrophils stimulated in vitro with beta-1,3-D-polyglucose derivatives. *Microbiol. Immunol.* 36:1173-1188, 1992.

72. Rasmussen, L.T., Fandrem, J. and Seljelid, R. Dynamics of blood components and peritoneal fluid during treatment of murine E. coli sepsis with beta-1,3-D-polyglucose derivatives. II. Interleukin 1, tumour necrosis factor, prostaglandin E2, and leukotriene B4. *Scand. J. Immunol.* 32:333-340,1990.

73. Rasmussen, L.T. and Seljelid, R. Dynamics of blood components and peritoneal fluid during treatment of murine E. coli sepsis with beta-1,3-D-polyglucose derivatives. I. Cells. *Scand. J. Immunol.* 32:321-331, 1990.

74. Rasmussen, L.T. and Seljelid, R. Novel immunomodulators with pronounced in vivo effects caused by stimulation of cytokine release. *J. Cell Biochem.* 46:60-68, 1991.

75. Rayyan, W. and Delville, J. [Effect of beta-1,3 glucan and other immunomodulators of microbial origin on experimental leprosy in mice]. *Acta Leprol.* 1:93-100, 1983.

76. Ronzio, R., *The Encyclopedia of Nutrition & Good Health*, Facts on File Inc., NY, NY, 1997.

77. Sakurai, T., Hashimoto, K., Suzuki, I., Ohno, N., Oikawa, S., Masuda, A. and Yadomae, T. Enhancement of murine alveolar macrophage functions by orally administered beta-glucan. *Int. J. Immunopharmacol.* 14:821-830, 1992.

78. Seljelid, R. Tumour regression after treatment with aminated beta 1-3D polyglucose is initiated by circulatory failure. *Scand. J. Immunol.* 29:181-192, 1989.

79. Sherwood, E.R., The role of macrophages in the antitumor activity of glucan. *Diss. Abstr. Int.*(Sci). 48:1263, 1987.

80. Sherwood, E.R., Williams, D.L. and Di Luzio, N.R. Comparison of the in vitro cytolytic effect of hepatic, splenic and peritoneal macrophages from glucan-treated mice on sarcoma M5076. *Methods Find. Exp. Clin. Pharmacol.* 8:157-161, 1986.

81. Sherwood, E.R., Williams, D.L. and Di Luzio, N.R. Glucan stimulates production of antitumor cytolytic/cytostatic factor(s) by macrophages. *J. Biol. Response. Mod.* 5:504-526, 1986.

82. Sherwood, E.R., Williams, D.L., McNamee, R.B., Jones, E.L., Browder, I.W. and Di Luzio, N.R. In vitro tumoricidal activity of resting and glucan-activated Kupffer cells. *J. Leukoc. Biol.* 42:69-75, 1987.

83. Slejelid, R. Macrophage activation. *Scand. J. Rheumatology* 76:67-72,1988.

84. Soltys, J., Benkova, M. and Boroskova, Z. Immunorestorative effect of glucan immunomodulator on guinea pigs with experimental ascariosis. *Vet. Immunol. Immunopathol.* 42:379-388, 1994.

85. Stewart, C.C., Valeriote, F.A. and Perez, C.A. Preliminary observations on the effect of glucan in combination with radiation and chemotherapy in four murine tumors. *Cancer Treat. Rep.* 62:1867-1872, 1978.

86. Takeda, Y., Yoshikai, Y., Ohga, S. and Nomoto, K. Augmentation of host defense against Listeria monocytogenes infection by oral administration with polysaccharide RBS (RON). *Int. J. Immunopharmacol.* 12:373-383, 1990.

87. Thompson, I.M., Spence, C.R., Lamm, D.L. and DiLuzio, N.R. Immunochemotherapy of bladder carcinoma with glucan and cyclophosphamide. *Am. J. Med. Sci.* 294:294-300, 1987.

88. Walinder, G., Arora, R.G., Bierke, P., Broome-Karlsson, A. and Svedenstal, B.M. Effects of glucan on the reticuloendothelial system and on the development of tumors in 90Sr-exposed mice. *Acta Oncol.* 31:461-467,1992.

89. Weiner, M. A., *Maximum Immunity*, Houghton Mifflin Company, Boston, 1986.

90. Williams, D., Sherwood, E.R., Browder, W., McNamee, R., Jones, E.R. and DiLuzio, N.R. Pre-clinical safety evaluation of soluble glucan. *Int. J. Immunopharmac.* 10:405-414, 1988.

91. Williams, D.L., Browder, I.W. and Di Luzio, N.R. Immunotherapeutic modification of Escherichia coli—induced experimental peritonitis and bacteremia by glucan. *Surgery* 93:448-454, 1983.

92. Williams, D.L. and Di Luzio, N.R. Glucan induced modification of experimental Staphylococcus aureus infection in normal, leukemic and immunosuppressed mice. *Adv. Exp. Med. Biol.* 121:291-306, 1979.

93. Williams, D.L. and Di Luzio, N.R. Glucan-induced modification of murine viral hepatitis. *Science* 208:67-69, 1980.

94. Williams, D.L., Sherwood, E.R., Browder, I.W., McNamee, R.B., Jones, E.L. and Di Luzio, N.R. The role of complement in glucan-induced protection against septic shock. *Circ. Shock.* 25:53-60, 1988.

95. Williams, D.L., Sherwood, E.R., Browder, I.W., McNamee, R.B., Jones, E.L., Rakinic, J. and Di Luzio, N.R. Effect of glucan on neutrophil dynamics and immune function in Escherichia coli peritonitis. *J. Surg. Res.* 44:54-61, 1988.

96. Williams, D.L., Sherwood, E.R., McNamee, R.B., Jones, E.L., Browder, I.W. and Di Luzio, N.R. Chemoimmunotherapy of experimental hepatic metastases. *Hepatology* 7:1296-1304, 1987.

97. Williams, D.L., Yaeger, R.G., Pretus, H.A., Browder, I.W., McNamee, R.B. and Jones, E.L. Immunization against Trypanosoma cruzi: adjuvant effect of glucan. *Int. J. Immunopharmacol.* 11:403-410, 1989.

98. Wyde, P. Beta-1,3-glucan activity in mice: intraperitoneal and oral applications. Baylor College of Medicine Research Report: 1989.(Abstract)

Appendix I

Conditions and descriptions

Following are descriptions of health conditions that are characterized by a weakened immune system. Finding ways to bolster immune function will help improve these conditions.

AIDS and HIV infection

AIDS (acquired immune deficiency syndrome) is a severe immune deficiency state due to an infection of the human immunodeficiency virus (HIV). The major methods of transmission of HIV are sexual contact, blood-to-blood contact (through blood transfusions or needle-sharing in drug addicts), and from woman to fetus. AIDS is not present in all persons infected with HIV. AIDS represents the end stage of the infection and severe depression of the immune system.

Bronchitis and pneumonia

Bronchitis refers to an infection or irritation of the bronchial tube, while pneumonia refers to infection or irritation of the lungs. Both are characterized by chills, fever, and chest pain. Pneumonia shows more signs of lung involvement (shallow breathing, cough, abnormal breath sounds, etc.). X-rays of patients with pneumonia show infiltration of fluid and lymph in the lungs. Of the two conditions, pneumonia is by far the more serious.

Cancer

Cancer is a complex condition characterized by an unrestrained growth of cells. Most malignant cancers develop in organs, such as the lungs, breasts, prostate, pancreas, colon, etc., but they may also develop in other tissues and spread. Standard medical treatment of malignancies can include surgery, chemotherapy, and radiation. Chemotherapy and radiation expose healthy cells, as well as cancer cells, to free-radical damage. The result is a great stress to antioxidant mechanisms and depletion of valuable antioxidant enzymes and nutrients.

Candidiasis

Candida overgrowth is now becoming recognized as a complex medical syndrome known as the yeast syndrome or chronic candidiasis. This overgrowth is believed to cause a wide variety of symptoms in virtually every system of the body. The gastrointestinal, genitourinary, endocrine, nervous, and immune systems are the most susceptible. Many illnesses can be traced to candida overgrowth.

Common cold

The common cold is caused by a variety of viruses that infect the oral and nasal passages and the sinuses. Symptoms of a cold are well-known: fever, headaches, nasal congestion, sore throat, or generalized malaise. Colds can be prevented by strengthening the immune system. Getting more than one or two colds a year, or having a cold that lasts more than four or five days are signs of a weakened immune system.

Ear infection (chronic otitis media)

An acute middle-ear infection (acute otitis media) is characterized by a sharp, stabbing, dull, and/or throbbing pain in the ear. The pain is due to inflammation, swelling, or infection of the middle ear. Acute ear infections are usually preceded by an upper respiratory infection or allergy. The organisms most commonly cultured from middle ear fluid during acute otitis media include *Streptococcus pneumoniae* (40 percent) and *Haemopilus influenzae* (25 percent). Chronic otitis media refers to a constant swelling of the middle ear and affects 20 to 40 percent of children under the age of six. They account for over 50 percent of all visits to pediatricians.

Hepatitis

A virus causes hepatitis in most instances. Viral types A, B, and C are the most common. Hepatitis A occurs sporadically or in epidemics, and is transmitted primarily through fecal contamination. Hepatitis B is transmitted through infected blood or blood products. It is occasionally transmitted through saliva and sexual secretions. Hepatitis C is primarily transmitted through blood transfusion. Acute viral hepatitis is characterized by loss of appetite, nausea, vomiting, fatigue, and other flu-like symptoms; fever; enlarged, tender liver; jaundice (yellowing of skin due to the increased level of bilirubin in the blood); dark urine; and elevated liver enzymes in the blood. Ten percent of hepatitis B and 10 to 40 percent of hepatitis C cases develop into chronic viral hepatitis forms. The symptomatology varies.

Herpes

The Herpes simplex virus (HSV) can produce a recurrent viral infection on virtually any area of skin or mucous membranes. The most common sites are around the mouth (cold sores) and the genitals. Herpes simplex 1 usually causes cold sores while the type 2 virus usually causes genital herpes. The rash in genital herpes is characterized by the appearance of single or multiple clusters of small blisters filled with a clear fluid on a reddened base. The blisters eventually burst. When they do, they leave small, painful ulcers that heal within ten to 21 days.

Infections

An infection refers to a colony of disease-causing organisms establishing a home within the body. Infections can be caused by viruses, bacteria, yeasts, and other microorganisms. The organisms actively reproduce and cause disease directly by damage to cells, or indirectly by releasing toxins. It is the function of the immune system to combat infections. Different aspects of the immune system deal with different microorganisms.

Parasites (intestinal)

A parasite is any organism living in or on any other living creature. When people refer to "intestinal parasites," most often they are loosely referring to single-celled organisms known as protozoa (such as giardia and amoeba). However, strictly speaking, all organisms in the intestinal tract are parasites, even health promoting bacteria such as *L. acidophilus*. Because of the seriousness of some untreated protozoan infection, see a doctor if you are experiencing symptoms of violent attacks of diarrhea, severe abdominal discomfort, and fever.

Periodontal disease and gingivitis

Periodontal disease is characterized by localized pain of the gum tissue, loose teeth, dental pockets, redness, swelling and/or pus, or jaw bone destruction. Periodontal disease usually begins as gingivitis, which is inflammation, redness, and/or bleeding of the gums. An estimated 80 to 90 percent of the American population has some degree of periodontal disease.

Sinus infection

An acute sinus infection is characterized by nasal congestion and discharge, fever, chills, frontal headache, and pain, tenderness, redness, and swelling over the involved sinus. A chronic infection may produce no symptoms other than mild postnasal discharge, a musty odor, or an unproductive cough. The most common predisposing factor in acute bacterial sinusitis is viral upper respiratory tract infection (e.g., the common cold). Allergies and other factors which interfere with normal protective mechanisms may precede the viral infection and, therefore, are also likely predisposing factors. Any factor which induces swelling and fluid retention of the mucous membranes of the sinuses may cause blockage or drainage. In this scenario, bacterial overgrowth occurs.

Appendix II

Other natural immune stimulators

Aloe vera

Out of more than 300 species of aloe, aloe vera is the most popular and medicinal variety. Aloe contains a variety of active constituents, including fatty acids, enzymes, amino acids, vitamins, and minerals. Mannan from aloe has been studied extensively as a positive immune enhancer. Aloe vera has a variety of uses: antibacterial, antifungal, antiviral, anti-inflammatory, and wound healing.

Beta-carotene/carotenoids

Beta-carotene is the most studied nutrient of a group of compounds known as carotenoids. These substances have extensive antioxidant capacity, making them ideal for immune system stimulation. Carotenoids are used to enhance immune function in conditions such as cancer. They have also been shown to benefit the cardiovascular system.

Coenzyme Q10

CoQ10 is a powerful antioxidant that works within the cells, providing energy and helping to metabolize fat and carbohydrates. CoQ10 helps bolster the immune system and can help protect against chemotherapy and radiation. In addition to stimulating the immune system, CoQ10 provides extensive benefit to the cardiovascular system.

Echinacea

This widely studied herb is used to treat the common cold, infections, low immune status, and cancer. Echinacea contains a wide range of active constituents that work on many different levels of immunity. Echinacea is believed to specifically stimulate T-cell activity.

Garlic

Population studies have shown that cultures that eat a lot of garlic have substantially reduced rates of cancer. Garlic has been shown to be an effective preventive and treatment method for cancer. In addition, garlic protects against bacteria, viruses, and fungi. As well as being a strong immune system stimulator, garlic also benefits the cardiovascular system.

Goldenseal

Goldenseal has often been referred to as "nature's antibiotic." The active component in goldenseal, berberine, demonstrates a broad range of antibiotic activity. In addition, berberine has been shown to increase blood flow to the spleen, an important immune-system organ.

Grape seed extract

A powerful antioxidant botanical, grape seed extract has been proven effective for wound healing and immune-system stimulation. Grape seed extract is most effective in the treatment of vein and capillary disorders such as diabetic retinopathy, macular degeneration, and varicose veins.

Green tea

Cultures that consume more green tea have far lower frequency of cancer and other diseases associated with a weakened immune system. Green tea is a potent antioxidant and protects against cancer.

Selenium

Recent studies have shown this important trace mineral helps prevent and treat some serious forms of cancer. Selenium is another natural antioxidant that can activate a positive immune-system response, stimulating the body's own healing capability.

Spleen and thymus glandular extracts

Glandular extracts operate on the premise that "like heals like." If you feed the body extract of the corresponding gland, the theory is that it will stimulate that gland and keep it operating effectively. Extracts of bovine spleen and thymus tissue have been shown to elicit a strong immune-system response. Thymus extracts are particularly used in cases of viral hepatitis, while spleen extracts are recommended for cancer prevention and treatment.

ACTIVATE YOUR IMMUNE SYSTEM

Vitamin C

This important nutrient has been widely studied for its antioxidant activity. It has been shown to stimulate a positive immune response. For more information on vitamin C, refer to Chapter Three.

Vitamin E

Another critical antioxidant nutrient, vitamin E serves many important purposes, including immune-system stimulation. Vitamin E has also been shown to benefit the cardiovascular system, as well as help alleviate menopausal symptoms.

Zinc

This antioxidant mineral stimulates the immune system by activating T-cells. Zinc supplementation has been shown to improve white cell counts and antibody production. In addition to being useful in the prevention and treatment of cancer, zinc plays a major role in tissue repair.

Appendix III

Resources

Web sites

www.healthy.net

www.impakt.com

www.immudyne.com

www.raysahelian.com

http://npjobs.com/aanp/links.htm

Organizations

American Association of Naturopathic Physicians
601 Valley Street, Suite 105
Seattle, WA 98109
Referral line (206) 298-0125

The American Osteopathic Association
142 E. Ontario St.
Chicago, IL 60611
(800) 621-1773

The American Botanical Council
P.O. Box 201660
Austin, TX 78720
(512) 331-8868, Fax (512) 331-1924

American College of Advancement in Medicine
P.O. Box 3427
Laguna Hills, CA 92654
(800) 532-3688, Fax (949) 455-9679

National Center for Homeopathy
801 N. Fairfax, Suite 306
Alexandria, VA 22314
(703) 548-7790, Fax (703) 548-7792

The Center for Mind/Body Medicine
5225 Connecticut Ave. NW, Suite 414
Washington, DC 20015
(202) 966-7338, Fax (202) 966-2589

Longevity Research Center
Ray Sahelian, M.D., Director
P.O. Box 12619
Marina Del Rey, CA 90295
(310) 821-2409

Index

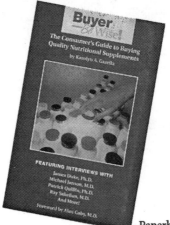

For a **free** catalog of
books and booklets
published and distributed
by IMPAKT Communications,
send the completed form to the address
below, or fax it to 1-920-434-8884.

IMPAKT Communications
P.O. Box 12496
Green Bay, WI 54307-2496

Please send me a FREE catalog!

FIRST NAME_____

LAST NAME_____

COMPANY (IF APPLICABLE)_____

MAILING ADDRESS_____

CITY_____ STATE _____ ZIP_____

PHONE _(____)_____

i M PAKT
IMPAKT Communications
www.impakt.com